To Nancy
from June.

1982

First two editions published under the
title *Notes for the Guidance of
Parents of Diabetic Children*
by J.W. Farquhar

THE
DIABETIC
CHILD

J.W. FARQUHAR MD, FRCPE

Professor, Department of Child Life and Health,
University of Edinburgh; Consultant Physician, The Royal
Hospital for Sick Children, Edinburgh

 CHURCHILL LIVINGSTONE
EDINBURGH LONDON MELBOURNE AND NEW YORK 1981

CHURCHILL LIVINGSTONE
Medical Division of Longman Group Limited

Distributed in the United States of America
by Churchill Livingstone Inc., 19 West 44th Street, New York,
N.Y. 10036, and by associated companies,
branches and representatives throughout
the world.

Third Edition 1981

First two editions published under
the title *Notes for the Guidance
of Parents of Diabetic Children*
by J.W. Farquhar

ISBN O 443 02193 7

British Library Cataloguing in Publication Data
Farquhar, James Watson
   The diabetic child.
   1. Diabetes in children
   I. Title
   618.9'24'62   RJ420.D5   80-41641

Printed in Singapore by Singapore Offset Printing Pte. Ltd.

CONTENTS

1. Just diagnosed? Here's good news! — 1
2. What has food to do with diabetes? — 8
3. All about insulin — 20
4. What about eating? — 37
5. Exercise — 49
6. How do we know treatment is correct? — 50
7. Short-term complications — 58
8. Going home — 66
9. The crystal ball — 69
10. Games diabetic children play — 76
11. Make your choice — 80
12. Diabetic hostels — 83
13. Your good health! — 84
14. Children's camps — 86
15. Travelling — 88
16. The family abroad — 92
17. A last word — 95
Appendix 1 Young diabetics — 97
Appendix 2 Carbohydrate exchange list — 100
Appendix 3 Emergency rations — 108
Index — 111

1. JUST DIAGNOSED? HERE'S GOOD NEWS!

If you are a parent reading this in hospital with the diagnosis 'diabetes' still ringing in your ears and filling your mind, then your child may at this moment look very ill — may even be unconscious. Most youngsters who get to hospital alive improve miraculously during the first few hours. They are likely to be looking around them by the second day and to be home after only one week. Take a look at Figure 1a, b, c and see for yourself. They will then live a normal life and should make progress at home, at school, at play and eventually at work.

And you? You will find in the first week that you *can* give the treatment and keep your child healthy so that he * becomes a healthy adult, a happy husband if the right girl comes along and a proud father if good diabetic care is continued[+]. You do not need to know all of this book in the next week, the next year or ever to have him looking really well. For these first few days *your* job is to be with him for as much time as the family can spare you so that you may reassure him about recovery and health. The doctors and nurses will provide all the technical care needed. Your turn will come in a day or two. In the meantime *smell* his breath. Can you smell something rather *sweet* like nail varnish

---

* For simplicity we shall use 'he, his, him' but read 'she, hers, her' where necessary.
[+] Assuming he is healthy otherwise

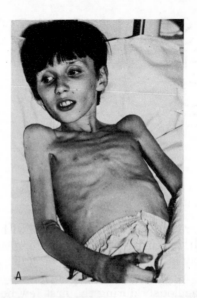

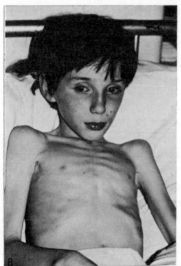
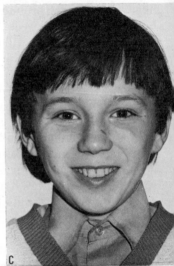

Fig.1 (a) On admission to hospital; (b) four hours after admission; (c) one year later. (Figs. 1a and b are reproduced by kind permission of Dr. Neil C. Fraser.)

remover? That smell is due to 'ketones' and the staff can produce some for you in a bottle so that you may familiarise yourself with the smell. It is a very important sign that a diabetic needs medical advice. Don't worry if you cannot smell it — you will be given a very easy test (p.51) which will show you if your child is excreting ketones in his urine.

Watch his breathing also. It may be very deep and almost sighing. This too is an important sign of the acute illness. He is trying to blow off through his lungs a severe acidity which has developed in his blood. I hope that you will never see it again but do remember it 'just in case'.

MESSAGE: he is going to be as fit as ever and much fitter than he has been recently. He can be NORMAL! NORMAL! NORMAL! except for his treatment.

If you would like to speak to a mother of a diabetic child, ask doctor or nurse to fix it.

What are they doing to him?

So there you are sitting by his bed-side or in the waiting-room and you would like to know what the doctors and nurses are doing to him.

If he was well enough to walk to his bed on admission and if he was fully conscious and not vomiting then he may be having only 2 or 3 little injections of the magic liquid 'insulin'. I shall shortly describe what that is. These alone will work wonders in the next 24 hours.

If however he was *carried* into the hospital or if he has been vomiting and is very dry then he is probably being given water containing various salts (glucose will be added later) from a plastic or glass container which is hanging above his bed. The fluid runs through a plastic tube which passes through a little skin puncture into a vein. This is painless and the fluid slowly corrects his problem when it is given along with insulin. This insulin is in clear liquid form. He may be receiving it very slowly through the same vein — pushed very very gently by a syringe which is driven by an electric motor. This system is usually discontinued in 1 or 2 days when he can drink and eat without vomiting. The punctured skin and vein heal almost at once.

Really big boys and girls (older teenagers) may have the water and salts solution to which insulin has already been added while some hospitals treat all children with injections of insulin repeated every hour. Don't worry about his not getting food or drink by mouth at this stage. The tube in his vein gives him all he needs and he will put on weight quickly when he goes home. Doctors call this system of feeding into a vein 'intravenous therapy' which simply means that his treatment is going straight into his blood stream. In hospital jargon it is an 'i.v.' or 'a drip'.

If he is very drowsy or unconscious and particularly if he has been vomiting, you may even see a fine plastic tube coming out of one nostril. It may be taped lightly to his face. This is used to reduce vomiting because in such circumstances there is a danger of vomit going back down the wrong way and choking him. It is not uncomfortable and it will be removed within a day or so in most cases.

There may also be other electrical equipment by his bedside to keep a check on his heart-rate and blood pressure. This is needed sometimes to help the staff choose the right treatment.

From time to time nurses will be noting his heart and respiratory rates, checking the amounts of fluid and insulin given and taking blood samples for important signs that he is returning to normal. Don't worry about all this activity. It is routine in these circumstances.

Why did he get diabetes?

First let me assure you that he has not got diabetes because of something that his parents have done or not done.

Perhaps it seems unbelievable to you that, in an age when hearts and kidneys can be transplanted, when many of the killing infections can be prevented or cured and when there are doctors specialised in deep-sea and outer-space medicine, we still do not know with certainty the *cause* of such a very common disease as diabetes. Thousands of research workers throughout the world have wrestled with this exceedingly complicated subject for much of this century. The scientific information about it would fill a library. The final break-through may be getting closer but we do not yet have the answer to the question 'why did he get diabetes?'

It is just as surprising, but a great deal more fortunate, that although we do not know the cause, we *do* know the treatment. Before 1921, the diagnosis of diabetes in child-hood meant certain rapid melting away and death. Now-adays Life Insurance Companies regard diabetics (*who have a doctor's certificate to say that they look after themselves very well*) almost as normal risks.

There are probably different kinds of diabetes but the symptoms (that is what the patient is complaining about) are caused in all of them by damage to a gland, weighing about 90g* in an adult, which lies close to the stomach. It is called the *pancreas* and it is a very complicated factory which makes many important chemicals concerned with regulating our supply and use of energy (food). In diabetics the tiny bits of this gland which make *insulin* are sick or dead. They have worn out slowly in middle aged and older people (particularly stout ones) who become diabetic but in children they are damaged by a sudden acute attack. Some very particular infections may play a part but there is almost certainly an inborn inherited factor which makes some children much likelier to get diabetes than others.

Without his personal factory for making insulin the diabetic cannot use sugar properly and it accumulates in the blood with very serious effects — but I shall tell you about that later.

* approximately 3 ounces

More good news

You are not alone. Not only does the hospital know exactly how you should look after him but so does your family doctor. Furthermore the hospital consultant will keep in regular contact with your family doctor.

Some hospitals have 'home care teams' which are trained to work with doctors and nurses in the community. They can correct many of the problems without your needing to come to hospital at all and are ready with helpful advice based on long experience. Some provide a telephone advice service.

In addition to the Health Service many countries have Diabetic Associations which raise money to provide advisory services, fund research, negotiate with government departments and help diabetic children by running summer camps and organising 'teach-ins' for their parents. The British Diabetic Association at 10 Queen Anne Street, London WIM OBD will be delighted to enrol you as a member and will give you the address of your nearest branch secretary. Membership entitles you to receive the B.D.A. newspaper *Balance* which is full of interesting articles.

Some areas also have Parents' Groups which can be quite encouraging since not only may they have interesting speakers but can exchange experiences with other parents. In Britain about 1 child in every 1000 under 16 years of age is diabetic so in a small town several of you are coping with the same problem and may be able to help each other.

It is more good news than bad news to say that in only a minority of families is more than one child diabetic although it certainly does happen. Even when one of identical twins becomes diabetic the other may remain normal. There is at least some reason for hope that within the next 10 years it may be possible to protect vulnerable children from the disorder. So don't fret about other children — it may never happen.

Beware of false news

In the next few weeks you may well be given false bad news. We all know how people are fascinated more by bad news than they are by good news! How many newspapers would be sold if they confined themselves to health, wealth and happiness? Watch your television tonight or listen to your radio for news — how much of it is good? Some people love to carry bad news and to watch the resulting dismay, fear, anxiety or doubt. Even mothers of diabetic children may spread alarm among others whose children are newly diabetic. That is why this book is going to tell you the truth about diabetes so far as doctors understand it in 1980.

Thus it is NOT TRUE that diabetic children get gangrene of their feet from ill-fitting shoes or from cutting toe-nails. It is NOT TRUE that they can go blind from wearing tight hats (not that many do nowadays), or bumping their heads. It is NOT TRUE that they should not play football or swim. It is NOT TRUE that diabetic girls often need to go into hospital for their periods. It is NOT TRUE that diabetic girls cannot have babies. It is NOT TRUE that diabetic children should avoid academic studies at school — and so on. If someone tells you an alarming story about childhood diabetics, don't lose sleep over it, ask your doctor if it's true.

On the other hand people pick up the strangest ideas about new treatments from newspapers, magazines, radio and television. I am regularly assured by parents that a cure has been found in the Amazonian forests or somewhere in central Africa. The press thrives on sensationalism so don't get too excited about 'cures' and even if something new is reliably reported on television, that does not mean that it can be applied immediately in the Health Service. We all know that Man has been to the Moon but there are no package deal holidays as yet on the Costa Luna!

2. WHAT HAS FOOD TO DO WITH DIABETES?

We are plagued nowadays with incessant talk about *energy* — its sources, its cost, its scarcity, its impending crisis and how we should save it. We need energy to light and heat our homes, to move our transport and to work our factories. We need it ourselves. 'He's full of energy', we say; or 'I seem to have no energy'.

A gas cooker uses gas for energy. It uses it to heat and cook. If there is no gas there are no smiles from the family. On the other hand we may have lots of gas flowing out of the burners but if we do not have a light (ignition) there will be a very nasty smell and we shall need to open all the windows if we are not going to go up in a loud bang!

The body is like that. If it does not get a flow of energy (as food) it can do nothing. On the other hand if it gets lots of energy as food but has no light (insulin) to convert it to activity and heat, then food builds up in the blood to dangerous levels. The body becomes very sick. It will certainly 'open its windows' by flushing sugar out through the kidneys in urine but this is not enough and the ambulance rushes the poor sick body off to hospital so that doctors can introduce insulin and burn off the excess.

Let us look very simply at food and how its energy is used to power the body.

Food

Most people who read this book will have enough to eat (very possibly too much) and will choose what they enjoy. Increasingly there is a move to simple, unrefined 'whole foods'.

Protein

Protein is a principal source of building material used by children for growth. The poor, stunted, swollen, dying children you see on posters appealing for help in famine areas of the world have had insufficient protein. Rich animal sources are eggs, bacon and ham, beef, veal, lamb, pork, liver, kidney, tripe, tongue, chicken, rabbit, fish and cheese. They are expensive and tend to be rationed by price so that they are unlikely to be eaten in excess. In practice therefore we seldom restrict their intake. Milk is an excellent source of protein but also contains 'sugar of milk' (lactose) and diabetics do need to measure it (we deal with this later, p.39).

Vegetarians in Britain get quite a lot of their protein from milk and eggs but the rest comes from vegetable sources such as peas, beans, nuts and grains.

Fat

Fat is a very rich source of energy. Animals accumulate it (and so do we unfortunately!) as a reserve to carry them through periods of starvation but it can be used too as a quick source of power. Meat and some fish contain it. Cream is fat and of course we use a lot (butter, margarine, edible oil or fat) in cooking, especially in frying. We have passed through 20 years when medical scientists have been very worried about animal fats as a possible cause of heart disease. If this is correct then diabetics would be wise to avoid them as much as possible since coronary thrombosis may be commoner in middle aged diabetics. Some distinguished nutritionists still believe an excess of animal fats to be dangerous but others are going off the idea. Since grilled food is often nicer than fried; since vegetable oil is often nicer than cooking fat and since some soft margarines may now be cheaper than butter

9

and just as flavoursome, it is no hardship to reduce animal fat intake 'just to be on the safe side'.

Carbohydrate

Carbohydrates are our cheapest readily available source of energy. They are commonly eaten as starches. Starches are available in flours, cereals, potatoes and other vegetables, pulses etc., and so we eat them as bread, biscuits, toast, rolls, pancakes, scones, buns, cakes, breakfast cereals, porridge, puddings, pasta and potatoes in all forms including chips and crisps. They are broken down by digestive juices (right from the mouth down through the small intestine) into the simple sugars which make up their constituent parts.

The sugars themselves of course are carbohydrates — much smaller units than starches, so they are more quickly absorbed from the gut and they are therefore faster fuels for energy. Every sportsman knows the name of one of these sugars — glucose. Fruit contains another — fructose. Milk contains yet another — lactose. Sugar cane and sugar beet contain another — sucrose. Whatever their form when they get into the blood from the intestine, they are all converted in human beings to glucose.

When glucose is taken by mouth it is almost immediately available in the blood for energy. When whole-meal bread is taken by mouth there is delay but it may be more sustaining since its energy is more slowly released as it is digested and absorbed. There are some other carbohydrates which Man cannot use at all and which pass through the bowel virtually unchanged. They provide what is now popularly known as 'fibre'. Some of these may even slow up the absorption of available sugars and because of this they have been used experimentally in treating diabetics.

The high energy content of sugar was well known to our grandparents when it was much cheaper than now. A little could be scattered on a reluctant fire to help it kindle. Putting a potato or a turnip in with the kindling materials would have had little effect! The body has the same problems. It undoubtedly finds it easier to deal with the quieter fire of a slowly climbing blood glucose level from digesting crude carbohydrate than with the blaze caused by a bag of chocolates.

Minerals and vitamins

Diabetics and non-diabetics alike need the same minerals and vitamins. Most children in this country now get enough but the doctor will advise you if he feels that some extras are needed.

Insulin and the effects of having none

Insulin is a very complicated substance. We cannot yet synthesise human insulin commercially although in 1980 germs have been taught to do so for us by genetic engineering. For the present we are fortunate in that insulin obtained from cattle and pigs is effective in human beings. In fact the insulin of pigs is so like that of man that humans accept it with little sign that their bodies recognise it to be foreign.

It is absolutely essential to the body and survival without it is impossible. It introduces energy (glucose) to the machinery of the body or, if the body is inactive, it may direct that the energy be converted into forms that can be stored. One of the most useful but sometimes most harmful conversions is changing glucose into fat.

We talk about the pancreas 'secreting' i.e. making insulin but it does not do so at the same pace all the time. It senses the arrival of food in the blood very quickly after its owner eats or drinks and sends out insulin into the blood stream to take care of it. In particular it senses the amount of glucose that has come in from starches or sugars and produces exactly the right amount of insulin to burn or store it. As the glucose level in the blood begins to fall, the pancreas slows the supply of insulin. It will immediately increase it to cope with the next snack or drink or meal. It has no time-switch turning it on at different times of day and it responds only to energy intake. So the rhythm is as shown in Figure 2a and b — food being followed by insulin.

If the body should make too much insulin (and sometimes it does make such a mistake) it will move too much glucose from the blood. The brain needs a certain minimum level of glucose on which to do its work and if the level gets too low it shows its displeasure by misbehaving. The person concerned feels tired, may become emotional, weak, drowsy and unconscious.

Fortunately the body is full of clever automatic correcting systems and several of these come into play when the blood glucose falls in response to insulin excess. The correcting systems open up the body's stores and release glucose into the blood.

The normal child's blood glucose level, like the adult's, is normally kept in a quite narrow range. Just like we measure flour in kilogrammes and milk in litres so we measure the blood glucose in millimoles per litre of blood and we abbreviate that to mmol/1. The range of normal may be taken as from 3.0 to 8.0 mmol/1. The figure is likely to be at the low end just before a meal and at the high end about one hour after a meal. Some doctors still use the previous system of units (milligrammes per 100 millilitres of blood — mg per 100 ml) and the same range in their terms is about 54 to 144 mg/100ml. In any case we are likely to be feeling hungry at the low end and satisfied at the top end.

If no insulin is available then there is no means of putting the accumulating glucose to use. He cannot use it and so his tissues are starved. He feels hungry at first but as the glucose steadily increases in his blood appetite often fails. A diabetic child at first diagnosis may have as much as 30 or 40 mmol of glucose per litre of blood (540 to 720 mg per 100 ml) or more. This has a very poisonous effect on all the body's tissues and a correcting device calls for water (thirst) so that the child has an almost constant craving to drink. Water will help him wash glucose out of the body through his kidneys. He passes

12

large volumes of urine often and it is full of glucose. It also contains ketones because when the body cannot use glucose for energy it begins to use fat instead. Ketones in the breath and urine are evidence of this — just as smoke coming from a chimney tells you that the house-holder has a fire in his grate.

These changes give rise to a linked chain of others. The body is starving because the food eaten cannot be used without insulin. Certain salts get lost in the urine and cause great muscular weakness. Acids gather up in the blood and another correcting device makes the child try to blow the acidity off by deep-breathing. In quite a short time inability to use energy, loss of water and poisoning with glucose and ketones produce drowsiness and coma. Before 1922 the child then died. The discovery of insulin makes death unnecessary provided that simple precautions are taken. Its skilful use as described on page 20 will bring most children back from the brink of disaster. From then on the whole modern aim of treatment in such children is to keep the level of blood glucose as near normal as possible for the rest of his life by the use of insulin, an ordered system of meals and healthy exercise. Failure to keep the blood glucose level normal leads, it is now believed, to nasty complications in 20 or more years.

Exercise, cold and weight- watching

Exercise is important to all animals and Man is no exception. Smoking, alcohol, over-eating, obesity and lack of exercise play big parts in causing serious illnesses and death in the developed countries.

Diabetic children need exercise not only to keep their muscles and heart fit but to help them burn up glucose and keep the blood level in the normal range. Parents of diabetic and of normal children alike should encourage exercise in safe conditions. Sustained exercise may be better than short sharp bursts. In Britain's variable climate the attraction of outdoor exercise varies but for diabetics it should be encouraged and parents should set good examples. Indoor

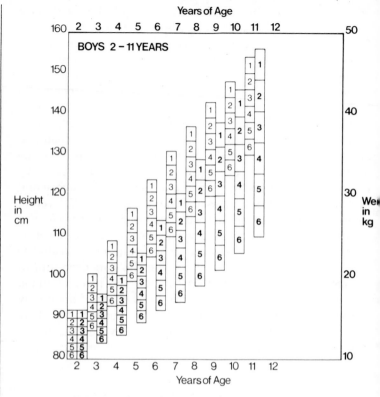

Fig. 2 Height and weight charts.

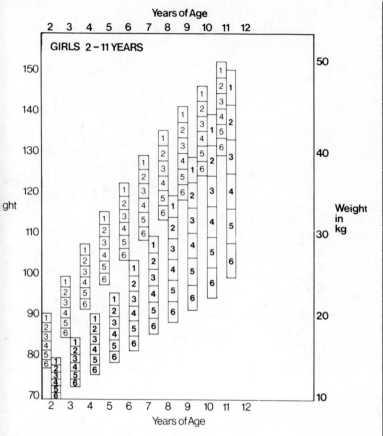

Fig. 2 (*cont'd.*)

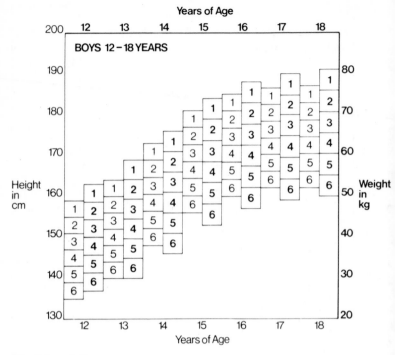

Fig. 2 (*cont'd.*)

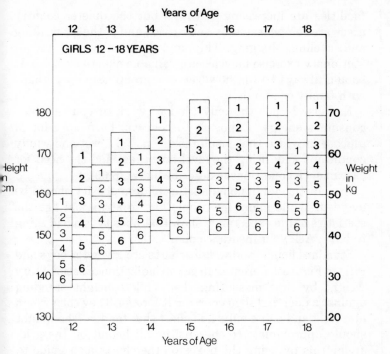

Fig. 2 (cont'd.)

facilities are increasing in towns but the quieter country areas are compensated by safer roads and paths for walking and cycling. Jogging, skipping, swimming and indoor stationary exercise bicycles are valuable aids to exercise. It should always be fun however — a group activity perhaps with family or friends.

Exercise is not the only kind of work of course which consumes energy. Exposure to cold can burn up a lot of glucose provided that insulin is given. Cold, wet and windy conditions may bring the level down fast and the need for care in such conditions is described later (p.60).

In diabetic and in non-diabetic children obesity should be avoided. While many fat people live to a ripe old age the statistics of life expectancy show that obesity is a bad thing to have. Ask your insurance man!

Standard height and weight charts are given for boys and girls in Figure 2. Parents can get an indication of satisfactory weight by first measuring their child's height standing against a door and then charting it for age. They then weigh him (vest and pants only) and chart that for age. The weight should approximate to the position of height on the grid. Judge this by using the boxes on the charts as a guide to position. Obese diabetics should attempt to cut food intake and increase the burning of energy on a regular basis.

Can we make the diabetic child normal?

The short answer is 'NO'.

Research activity continues throughout the world on means of providing diabetics with a replacement pancreas (transplanted human or man-made) and success is likely — but the cost cannot be predicted.

We can, however, give the diabetic child an almost normal childhood. Indeed, we can have him indistinguishable in classroom, playing-field and street from the other children who do not have diabetes. He can be happy, successful and popular. He can become an international footballer, a champion runner, a doctor, a baker, a nurse, a farmer. He will however need insulin and it is its administration which makes him different — first in the way he gets it, and secondly in the way it dictates his activities.

3. ALL ABOUT INSULIN

The difference between an average day for a diabetic child and for a non-diabetic one will now become clear. This section on the diabetic child begins with *insulin* whereas that on the normal child began with *food*. The diabetic child's pancreas cannot respond adequately* to food and to the resulting rise in blood glucose level. His treatment is *the replacement of insulin*. All other treatment follows from that.

The insulin obtained from the pancreases of cattle and pigs is a clear liquid. It is known as *soluble insulin* (in North America it may be called *regular insulin*). Unfortunately it cannot be taken by mouth since it is destroyed by the digestive juices and it must be given by injection into the fatty material beneath the skin. From there it gets into the blood and helps the body use its fuel (especially the carbohydrate) for work or to store it for later use. It has no power of its own to come into the blood just at the right time when food is eaten and there are very few diabetic adults, let alone diabetic children, who are willing to give themselves an injection every time they eat or drink.

And yet soluble insulin is most effective for only 2 or 3 hours after injection and then fades out. Obviously we cannot eat all our day's food in the morning when the insulin injection is given. So in the early years after insulin was discovered diabetics did need to have several injections each day. Then someone discovered how to prepare insulin in such

* Some function is left but it fades out after some attempted come-back.

20

a way that it was slowly released from the injection site. This made it possible to control diabetes with only *one injection per day* given just before breakfast. Since then the insulin manufacturers have prepared it in several different ways so that they are released at different rates into the blood. There are now many of them made by different firms in the world and to describe them all here would only be confusing. Your own clinic or family doctor can tell you what is used most in your community. The preparations can be classified very broadly as:

Short-acting	Up to 6 hours
Medium-acting	Up to 12-16 hours
Long-acting	Up to 30 hours

(The times are approximate and depend in part on the patient)

Few doctors now use long-acting insulins for children and indeed they are no longer used to the same extent even in adults.

Are insulin injections as good as a pancreas?

No, they are not. Remember that the pancreas produces spurts of insulin to deal with each intake of food or drink energy (Fig. 3a). A morning injection on the other hand, to change my previous analogy from gas-cookers for a moment, opens wide the body's furnace-doors to receive and deal with food taken during the next few hours (Fig. 3b). They are however self-closing doors and the gap through which to shovel the arriving food energy narrows steadily. This makes it necessary to control the amount of food arriving in the furnace room or it will pile up and choke everything. In terms of meals therefore the day's food must be spaced and measured so that it gets through the narrowing doors without causing trouble. It is just as true to say that if the doors of the body's furnace are left open and no fuel is put in — the fires will go out (hypoglycaemia).

21

NORMAL CHILD

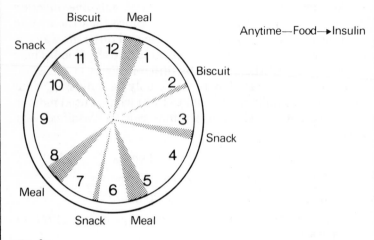

Anytime—Food—►Insulin

Fig. 3a

DIABETIC CHILD: Once daily insulin

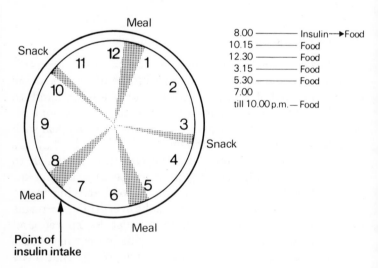

8.00	Insulin—►Food
10.15	Food
12.30	Food
3.15	Food
5.30	Food
7.00	
till 10.00 p.m. — Food	

Point of insulin intake

Fig. 3b

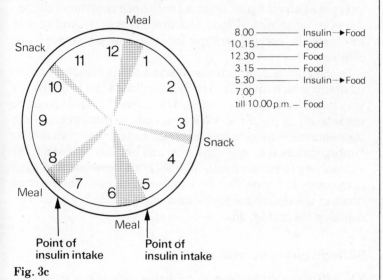

DIABETIC CHILD: Twice daily insulin

8.00 ——————— Insulin→Food
10.15 ——————— Food
12.30 ——————— Food
3.15 ——————— Food
5.30 ——————— Insulin→Food
7.00
till 10.00 p.m. — Food

Point of insulin intake

Point of insulin intake

Fig. 3c

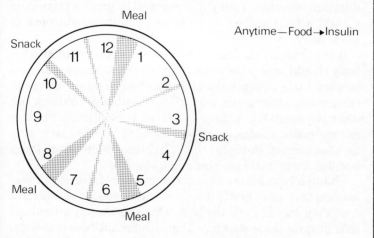

DIABETIC CHILD: Continuous variable flow-rate insulin

Anytime—Food→Insulin

Fig. 3d

Obviously there is no reason why more insulin cannot be injected at about 5 p.m. (Fig. 3c) to re-open the doors fully for the evening intake of food and drink energy — and this is what we do except perhaps in very new or very young children.

In the last year or two there have been successful experiments in which diabetics receive insulin all the time from a very small battery-operated electric pump. This pump can be made to inject insulin at varying speeds so that it can mimic the pancreas — more insulin at meals and less between meals. Unfortunately it is still expensive and has not yet been tried extensively in children although we have experimented with it in some. It is one way by which we can open the furnace doors at the right time and wide enough to take in the energy reaching them (Fig. 3d).

Different makes of insulin

You will probably find that your diabetic clinic has selected 2 or 3 insulins from the available range so that the staff become thoroughly familiar with them. You will be told the average duration of action. Your child may well be given a mixture of a short-acting and an intermediate-acting insulin once or twice daily.

It is obviously desirable that any injection going into the body should be as pure as possible and that it should cause no or very little adverse reaction (the body is very clever at recognising what is not part of itself and tries to throw out what is foreign e.g. kidney and heart transplants). For this reason many clinics, my own included, prefer very pure insulins derived from pigs to those derived from cattle. Purer insulins from cattle are now available.

Children have longer lives and many more injections ahead of them than have newly diagnosed adults and it seems right that they should have the best. This is perhaps particularly true of girls since we know that insulin antibodies can get from a pregnant woman to the baby in her womb. There is no good evidence that they can harm the baby but perhaps we should not risk it.

I have discussed pork (pig) insulins with well-informed physicians of the Jewish and Islamic religions and I understand that there is no objection to their use since the materials are very highly purified and have theoretical advantages over beef insulins or pork/beef insulin mixtures. Similarly, Hindus may have no objection to the use of beef insulin. My own clinic uses only highly purified short and intermediate-acting insulins (e.g. soluble and isophane) in combination. They can be mixed in the same syringe.

When to give insulin injections

In Britain it is customary to give an injection of insulin in the morning about 15 minutes before breakfast so that it will get into the blood and open the doors in time to deal with a carbohydrate (cereal) breakfast. *Mealtime dictates injection time*. The injected mixture will be such that it will keep the doors wide enough open to cope with meals through the rest of the morning and afternoon. Older children are probably better if given another before the evening meal but again here *mealtime dictates injection time*.

Now, if you are living in some other country with an entirely different system of meal times and meal contents your doctor may have some other system of injection times. Since *mealtime dictates injection time* it would be crazy to stick to British injection times for Sudanese mealtimes and meals. Your child should be an Iraqi, a Sudanese, a Malaysian or whatever his community is — and not a foreigner in his own land. You and your doctor will know when the main meals are taken and especially when the main load of carboydrate is taken. The injection times and the insulin mixtures are then given at the correct times to deal with them (See Fig. 3).

Strengths of insulin

Just as butter is measured in pounds or kilogrammes and petrol in gallons or litres, so insulin is measured in *units*. Depending upon its 'strength' each millilitre (ml*) of insulin contains either 40 or 80 units. Soluble insulin is the only one available at a strength of 20 units in each ml. Each strength of each kind of insulin has its own colours on the packet or label along with the strength in bold figures 20, 40 or 80. Note only the colours on the packets and labels of *your* child's insulin so that you do not get confused and always note also the strength 20, 40 or 80. *This is most important* if serious mistakes are to be avoided.[+]

In order to reduce the confusion which arises out of having several different strengths of insulin, some countries (North America particularly) have produced a new strength, i.e. 100 units in each ml. We conducted the British trial of this new strength in our hospital and believed it to be a great advance provided that the other strengths were no longer made. There are arguments for and against such a change but the British Diabetic Association is trying to have it introduced. It is a slow matter, however, because many diabetics would rather have the strength they have always used and the manufacturers of course are quite happy to keep on producing these original strengths. Indeed some maintain that so much insulin would be wasted in the production of 100 unit/ml that the total available for the world's population of diabetics might be reduced.

Storage of insulin

The manufacturers advise that all the insulins should be kept in a refrigerator but *never* in the freeze-box or in a deep freeze. *Don't* rush off and buy a refrigerator. A cool larder is perfectly adequate, provided that you do not store too much

* You are not going to measure insulin in teaspoonfuls but a plastic spoon for medicines holds 5 millilitres

[+] Some manufacturers recently abandoned colour coding.

insulin in it for too long. Your chemist's shop will look after it carefully and you need only have what will last you for a few weeks.

On the other hand if you are caring for your child in a country which has very hot seasons or where there is some danger of insulin being exposed in the open to the direct heat of the sun during transit, then you must be careful. At the following temperatures potency of insulin cannot be guaranteed beyond the periods given.

Temperature of store	Months of acceptable shelf-life	
°C	Soluble insulin	Intermediate insulin
30	13	11
40	3	1.5
45	1.5	0.6

It is necessary therefore in such climates that insulin be kept cool from arrival in the country until use.

Make and expiry date of insulin

Try always to get insulin that is made by the same manufacturer because they can vary a little bit. Note the expiry date on the label and do not use the insulin if it is older than the deadline. Note also the batch number in the book that you will be keeping so that your doctor can look at the relationship between this and any change of diabetic control which your child may show.

The syringe

A special glass syringe is available free through the National Health Service and is known as the BS1619 Standard Insulin Syringe (Fig. 4). Always refuse any other except a disposable plastic model of it. *It is dangerous to use any other syringe.*

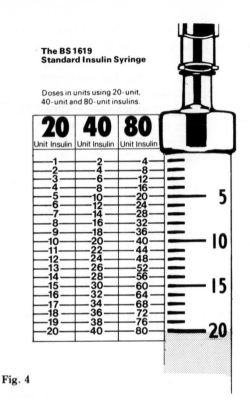

The BS 1619
Standard Insulin Syringe

Doses in units using 20-unit,
40-unit and 80-unit insulins.

20 Unit Insulin	40 Unit Insulin	80 Unit Insulin
1	2	4
2	4	8
3	6	12
4	8	16
5	10	20
6	12	24
7	14	28
8	16	32
9	18	36
10	20	40
11	22	44
12	24	48
13	26	52
14	28	56
15	30	60
16	32	64
17	34	68
18	36	72
19	38	76
20	40	80

Fig. 4

Serious mistakes have been made when chemists' shops and even hospitals have offered others as being 'just as good'. There is nothing anything like as good. Your doctor will prescribe two of them. Make sure that they have BS1619 clearly marked on them. Such syringes come in two sizes (1 ml and 2 ml) depending on the amount of insulin to be given. If you break one, get a prescription for another so that you always have the two which are required. This is so that you are never in the position where you break one some morning and have no replacement immediately available.

The BS1619 contains 20 units in 1 ml (ml, by the way, stands for millilitre or one-thousandth part of one litre) but it will only do so when you use soluble insulin at a strength of 20 units in one ml. To make the injections small we normally use insulin that is twice as strong (40 units in one ml) or even four times as strong (80 units in one ml). Putting it another way, if you use 40 units/ml insulin you need only half the volume and if you use 80 units/ml you need only one quarter the volume needed with 20 units/ml soluble insulin. Now read that through again looking at Figure 4. See how the 20 on the syringe is 20 units at 20 strength, 40 units at 40 strength and 80 units at 80 strength. Similarly, 16 units at 80 strength is only 4 on the syringe and 16 units at 40 strength is only 8 on the syringe. Got it?

Try another example. Someone's child needs 12 units of insulin. If the parents are using 20 units/ml strength, then they draw the plunger or piston gently up to 12. If they are using 40 units/ml insulin, which is twice as strong, they need only half as much so they draw the insulin up to 6. If they are using 80 units/ml insulin, which is four times as strong, they need only one quarter as much as with the 20 units/ml insulin and they draw it up to 3. At this point let me say, 'Don't panic!' The staff will go over and over and over it with you until you are absolutely sure of what you are doing. The dose does not vary much from day to day once treatment is well established.

Glass syringes are sterilised by boiling them in a small pan — the boiling kills off the germs. Ideally this should be done before each use of the syringe, but provided that they are always being used for the same patient they can be boiled once or twice a week and kept in alcohol for the rest of the time. A special blue spirit-proof plastic case is made by the Hypoguard firm (Hypoguard Limited, 49 Grimston Lane, Trimley, Ipswich, Suffolk) and can be prescribed on the National Health Service by your doctor. (At present you must pay for the thing to stand it in but a blob of kiddies' 'plasticine' makes a good substitute.) The case is filled with *industrial methylated spirit* for which you need your doctor's prescription. Neither ordinary methylated spirit from the hardware shop nor surgical spirit are as good. Take the syringe out of the case, shake off the drops of spirit, suck the plunger up and down a few times to get rid of what is inside, blow the spirit out of the syringe and you are ready to draw up and inject the insulin. After you have given the injection draw spirit up and down a few times into the barrel, then squirt it out and pop the lot into the spirit and screw it down. Both boiling and storage in industrial methylated spirit should be shown to you while your child is in hospital.

Patients living outside Britain may buy re-usable needles which should be sterilised and stored with the syringe. British child patients get free supplies of disposable ones.

Disposable and sterile plastic insulin syringes are available but cannot be prescribed free by the National Health Service. They are very good (some makes are better than others) and they do save time and bother in sterilising and storing glass ones. They are remarkably inexpensive — about the cost of two cigarettes — and smokers could improve their health by buying disposable syringes instead! Some clinics such as ours sell them to parents at virtually cost price. We know that for some years now parents and adult diabetics have been using the same plastic syringe several times before disposing of it — for up to 3 days perhaps. We know from experiments conducted here that these plastic syringes pick up germs even inside them during the first injection and we advised against their being reused. Recent practical experience in Britain and in the U.S.A. however suggest that the risk of their causing infection is very small if careful precautions are taken. These are that the syringe should be cleanly handled and that after use it should be slipped carefully back into its tube or packet and placed in the domestic refrigerator until it is next needed. In this way, according to the reports, the same plastic syringe may be used for 3 days. I do not recommend the practice but these reports state that it is widely used and causes no problems.

The needle

British diabetic children, under 16 years of age, are entitled to free sterile disposable needles which can be obtained from the hospital clinic. The child should have a fresh needle for each injection. Please obtain a drum from your hospital into which you drop each needle (and disposable syringe too if you like) after use. When it is full take it back to the hospital for special disposal. This practice prevents the spread of serious infections.

Giving insulin injections

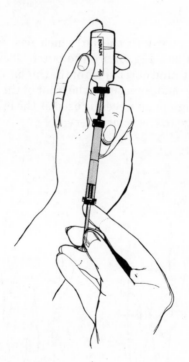

Fig. 5

Drawing up the insulin

With all insulins it is safer to roll the little bottle a few times between the palms to mix the insulin immediately before drawing up the dose. *Never* take the rubber cap off. Clean it with spirit. Stick the needle through the cap and inject the same amount of air as the amount of insulin you require. Then suck the insulin into the syringe. Hold it upside down with the little bottle of insulin on top with the needle still in it (Fig. 5) and squeeze the air bubbles from the syringe into the bottle. Adjust the plunger of the syringe to the correct mark. When children are learning to do this for themselves the dose should always be checked by a responsible person.

Sites for injection

Insulin is injected into the fat which lies below the skin. Suitable sites (see Fig. 6) are the outer sides of the upper arms, the fronts and outer sides of the thighs, the upper parts of the buttocks and sometimes the front of the abdomen. The back of the thigh must never be used as the injection may do serious damage to the sciatic nerve.

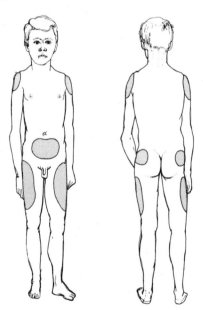

Fig. 6

It is important to keep changing the injection sites so that a separate place is used each day of the week, or alternatively the same part of the body is used for a week before moving on to another site. The important thing is to keep moving round in a set routine. By doing this you may reduce the risk of the ugly wasting or swelling of fat at the injection sites which afflicts some children.

Giving the injection

Clean the skin with industrial methylated spirit and cotton wool or, if you wish to buy them, with disposable swabs. Stretch the skin a little with the fingers. Push the needle of the loaded syringe obliquely into the skin so that the point passes quite through it and into the fat beneath it (Fig. 7). If you inject *into* the skin instead of below it there will be increased discomfort and possibly less satisfactory control. The quicker the action the less uncomfortable it will be. Press home the piston to inject the insulin. The technique will probably be practised first on an orange but since your child is likely to need two or three injections daily during the first few days you will see it done and then be able to do it yourself. Even some 5-year-olds can do it very soon and all children should be encouraged (but never forced) to do it as soon as possible.

Some children prefer to use the Palmer 'injector' (the word gun sometimes frightens nervous children so that they will not take to using it). The loaded syringe and needle are inserted into the carriage of the injector. The injector's guard is then pressed against the skin and on squeezing the trigger the syringe moves quickly forward and the needle passes through the skin. The piston of the syringe is then pressed home and the injection is over. The method has the advantages that the injector does everything very efficiently. You need not stretch the skin nor judge the angle of the injection nor even decide its depth, and the older diabetic child can inject himself with it using either his right or left hand. Some

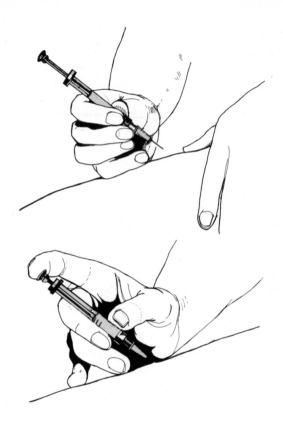

Fig. 7

parents have suggested that the gun should be used from the start as the child may accept it as part of routine treatment and get quickly used to it, whereas if it is offered later as an alternative he may fear and refuse it. Some disposable syringes jump out of the carriage during injection. This can be prevented by a few twists of elastic band. If you want to start using the Palmer injector in hospital under supervision, please ask the sister in charge if she has one and if you may try it. If she has none, you can write to the manufacturer (Palmer Injectors Limited, 166 Buchanan Street, Glasgow G1 2LW). The usual needle may be too short, so use a longer one of the same width to get the point through the skin. Adjust the guard.

The 'Hypoguard' (made by the same firm as makes the spirit-proof case and the Hypocount glucose monitor) is another aid to injection and requires the same sterilising technique as the syringe itself. It is simply one hollow metal tube within another, so arranged that the needle is hidden. When firmly held against the skin, pressure on the syringe component overcomes a little catch and the needle quickly enters the stretched skin at an appropriate angle and to an appropriate depth. The piston is then pressed home to deliver the insulin.

Regularly and carefully examine glass syringes. Leakage may take place sometimes at the junction with the needle or occasionally insulin may leak past the piston into the upper portion of the syringe and so escape injection. Loss of insulin in this way will upset the control of the patient's diabetes and such a syringe must be discarded and replaced. The dose of insulin varies very widely. It is usually high at first and may then fall during the first few months of treatment. Sometimes the child may need none for a short period but it will almost certainly be needed again later. The dose usually increases around the time of sexual development. Do not be anxious about the size of your child's insulin dose in relation to the amount of insulin which other mothers at the clinic may be giving to their children to exert the same good control. We have very little idea why some may need 10 units and others 100 or more. One explanation offered is that because the insulin you use is not human but comes from animals, humans destroy more or less of it because it is 'foreign' and so a bigger dose is needed to do the same amount of good. Don't worry about it, big doses are little more troublesome than small ones. The use of pork insulin from first diagnosis may help keep the dose smaller.

For some years now there has been available an injector powered either by a spring or, more conveniently, by a gas bulb, which does not involve pushing a needle through the skin. It expels the insulin with such force that the jet goes through the skin into the underlying fat. It is very costly and must of course be purchased privately. The British Diabetic Association has cautioned the public against rushing to buy it. There is a little concern still as to whether it might damage the skin and whether all the insulin goes through or whether some bounces off. Furthermore it is obvious that such injectors work by driving the insulin with such velocity that the jet is by itself a virtual needle. It remains an interesting development for those who can afford it.

Will he always need insulin injections?

The only effective treatment for childhood diabetes is insulin and the only method of giving it is by injection. The development of mini-pumps to give it may improve its efficiency and reduce the number of injections. Very rarely indeed cases are reported where childhood diabetes clears up, perhaps for ever. More commonly there is a short spell after first diagnosis and treatment when the insulin needs fall steadily and it may be possible to stop injections for a time. This may or may not be wise since the pancreas almost always becomes exhausted and insulin injections are seen to keep the child healthier and happier.

You will have heard that diabetes can be treated by swallowing tablets and sometimes people think that these are insulin tablets. They are quite unrelated to insulin but they can help those with residual insulin-making cells in their pancreas. Such people are usually middle aged or elderly. Children do not respond satisfactorily to them except in unusual cases — nor will they do so when they become middle aged or elderly people. The pancreas has been too heavily damaged and it has nothing left to give.

4. WHAT ABOUT EATING?

Since our system of injecting insulin once or twice daily does not mimic the true behaviour of the pancreas and of insulin in the human body the diabetic child's meals need to be gently modified both in their content and in their timing. This led years ago to the use of the word *diet* in relation to diabetic management. *The Oxford Dictionary* defines it as 'way of feeding; prescribed course of food, regimen; one's habitual food'. In order that a child's life may be as normal and as free as possible I prefer the meaning 'one's habitual food' and yet a measure of control is undoubtedly needed. It should be as unobtrusive as possible.

Few of us ordinary people ask mother or wife, 'What's our diet tonight?' The very word 'diet' for many of us implies some kind of special cooking concerned with illness. Most of us surely say, 'That smells good! What's for dinner?' Whatever it is, it should be for the diabetic member of the family too wherever possible, i.e. there should be one meal — the family meal. In saying this, however, we know that too many normal families eat in an unhealthy way. Doctors and other scientists have been studying food very closely in recent years. They still don't know all the answers as to its effect on health but they have some facts and some strong suspicions backed by evidence. Let me remind you again about some of these. Doctors and insurance men know, for example, that overweight people on average don't live as long as normal weight people. (Of course, lots of fat people do live to a ripe old age and thin ones may die young.) Fat people are fat because they *eat too much* — even if it is really less than the very thin man next door it is too much *for them*. They get fat because they eat, in particular, *too much carbo-*

hydrate for them and you know what carbohydrates are. Very many fat people are fat because they are *always nibbling carbohydrates* — eating between meals, a leftover piece of toast here, a biscuit there, a piece of chocolate and cups of tea or coffee with sugar. Doctors are still uncertain about the exact cause of coronary thrombosis ('heart attacks') in both diabetics and non-diabetics. Overweight diabetics are at greater risk. The kind of sugar you keep in your kitchen and which is used also to make sweets probably has, like smoking, a good deal to do with thrombosis if taken in excess. So may animal fats like cream, butter, suet and dripping. Vegetable oils and soft margarines which claim on the container to be 'high in polyunsaturates' are popular for cooking and spreading and may be started in childhood. They may even in some way protect the blood vessels from harm.

So good meals for *all* of us, diabetic or not, will get our weight into the normal range for our height (p.18) and keep it there. They should be well spaced out and we should not nibble in between them. We should take as little sugar as possible in or on our food. We may use corn oil in our frying and chip pans, and we shall probably find one of the soft spreading margarines to be a palatable and less expensive substitute for butter. Stop smoking, cut back on the beer if you are overweight for height, get a large dog, take it for long walks and let *it*, not *you*, eat the scraps. You will feel much better.

Similar simple rules and patterns of eating are best for diabetic eating. With enough insulin diabetic children can *survive* almost any kind of food. Parents surely want more than survival alone for them — they want an assured normal healthy future as well. That is why we apply to diabetic children the simple eating rules described above and in order to stress the diabetic child's normality we shall call the system not a diet but the Good Food System (GFS).

The good food system

This system is easy to understand and to use and makes

excellent control possible without being burdensome to patient, parent or family. The child takes protein and fat freely at meals (they are generally rationed by cost or taste).

Protein is available as meat and fish of all kinds. The meat includes bacon, offal, chicken and rabbit. Eggs and cheese are also excellent sources but milk cannot be freely given because it is rich in its own sugar known as lactose. You will find milk in the 'Exchange List' (p.102) and your child will of course get it (about 1 pint or 560 ml per day).

Fats are discussed above (p.9). He is allowed as much carbohydrate as he needs in the day. It is given in fairly even amounts at regular intervals but it can be as varied as required.

During your child's first admission to hospital you will be taught how to prepare his meals and in some hospitals (particularly children's hospitals or units) you may be able to stay with him if space exists. This is a good thing because you can then choose and perhaps even make his meals and you will be much more confident about your ability to look after him. He will probably be allowed home as soon as you have learned about his care since many doctors prefer to discharge such patients early even if the children are still passing glucose in their urine. Our average duration of stay in first admissions is 6 to 7 days for control and education. The finishing touches to good control are best done under home conditions. Where the hospital has no accommodation for mothers you may try to live nearby for a few days in order to get to hospital in time to give the insulin injection. The Royal Hospital for Sick Children, Edinburgh, has a Home Nursing Care team with special expertise in diabetes which furthers the parent's education actually in the home, advising about meals, etc., in the mother's own kitchen. This makes earlier discharge possible. It also gives the mother the chance to discuss in the privacy of her home such other matters as may be worrying her. Other hospitals may provide a similar service or the area may have special nurses trained to provide it. Home support is very welcome at this early stage but it is withdrawn as soon as possible so that the parent learns to take personal responsibility. It is always available of course at the end of a telephone when required.

Now for some details of the GFS. Look first at the British Diabetic Association (BDA) Exchange List (p.101). You will need diabetic scales. These are inexpensive little things which some but not all hospitals may arrange to lend to you for as long as they are required. With experience you can judge the food value with sufficient accuracy by eye or with a spoon.

The system will simply state that a certain number of 'exchanges' should be taken at each meal and the meals themselves should be equally spaced. For example a day's exchange intake in Britain might be scheduled as follows:

			Exchanges
8.00 a.m.	Breakfast		3
10.30 a.m.	Snack		2
12.30 p.m.	Lunch		4
3.00 p.m.	Snack		2
5.00 p.m.	Evening meal		4
7.00 − 10.00 p.m.	Snack		2
		Total	17

Meals in hospital may not be given at these times because they must fit in with other hospital activities. This is another good reason for getting the child home as soon as you are able to look after him. Similarly, they may not be precisely at these times at school and if they are too unevenly spaced, then you should ask for help at the clinic or from the school doctor or nurse.

Notice how we avoid giving a much bigger than usual carbohydrate meal at any time. It would be all wrong to let the diabetic have 7 or 8 exchanges at 5 p.m. when he has much less at other times. It could be done but he would almost certainly need a second injection of insulin just before it.

Let us look at a sample breakfast. We have given only 3

exchanges because children are often least hungry then. Set up your diabetic scales and if the marker is not reading 'O' on the scale ask how to adjust it. Take a breakfast cereal such as cornflakes (not one of the sugary or sticky cereals) and measure out 15 grams*. This is one of his three exchanges. He can have 30 grams if he likes but that would be two exchanges and he would have only one left. With the remainder he can have bread, toast or a bread roll (20 g of bread roll = 1 exchange) and milk (175 ml)+ and of course he can have butter, diabetic marmalade or jam (non-diabetic makes need to be included in the exchanges), eggs, bacon, fish, cheese or any other fat or protein food. He can have porridge if he likes but this would have to be included in his 3 exchanges so that you would have to find out what one exchange of porridge oats looks like in terms of tablespoons or ladles of the thickness of porridge which you usually make.

The midday meal is just as easy. Small amounts of soup need not be measured and, of course, clear soups and tomato juice may be taken as freely as wished. There are 4 exchanges to use. He may have unlimited amounts of meat, fish, cheese, eggs, green vegetables and salad, etc. Of his exchanges one might be potato (60 g) but he could have 2 exchanges (120 g) if he likes it, or indeed he could use all his exchanges as potato but this sounds rather an uninteresting meal. Peas or beans (60 g) would be another exchange and the remaining exchanges can be used for bread or for pudding. One plain individual piece of ice-cream is one exchange but he could have fruit or rice, sago, tapioca, etc. Note again that these are given as dry weights and you will have to work out how much pudding they make. The nurse visiting your home or the dietician at the clinic should be able to show you how.

You will have got the idea by now and so we shall not detail the evening meal. The 'snacks' can be protein and fat plus anything that makes 2 exchanges. Since our emphasis is on

* Weights are being expressed in metric terms. About 30 grams = 1 oz, 15 grams = ½ oz, 20 grams = ⅔ oz, etc. The use of the word grams under these circumstances refers to the actual weight of the food and not to its carbohydrate content.
+ 175 ml = ⅓ pint, 525 ml = 1 pint.

enjoying a normal life, continue whatever system of lunch he had before his diabetes was discovered. If at that time he came home for lunch let him do that now. If he took packed lunch to school, do that by packing the right number of exchanges. If he took school lunch, let him have it again but he should judge his bread, peas, beans, potatoes, etc. by eye and take the right amount of fresh fruit or biscuits and cheese to replace the common sweet, starchy puddings that tend to be part of school menus.

Other foods which are freely allowed

The following foods need not be measured:

Sprouts, cabbage, cauliflower, broccoli, french beans, runner beans, spinach, celery, artichokes, asparagus, marrow, mushrooms, onions, turnip, swede, small portions of carrots and leeks.

Lettuce, watercress, mustard and cress, chicory, radishes, cucumber, parsley, mint, chives, tomatoes, small amounts of beetroot.

Blackberries, blackcurrants, half grapefruit, loganberries, stewed gooseberries, red currants, lemons, rhubarb (sweetening must be non-sugar), olives, avocado pear.

Tea, coffee, clear soup, bovril, oxo, marmite, salt, pepper, mustard, herbs, spices, worcester sauce, pickles in vinegar.

You will find in the shops diabetic foodstuffs such as fruit juices and cordials, marmalades and jams as well as sweets which need not be counted as exchanges. The hospital dietician, your local chemist or grocer or the mothers of other diabetic children recommended to you at the clinic can keep you informed of these. Boots have a wide selection. Remember, however, that some are rich in non-carbohydrate energy (calories) and cannot be used in 'slimming' diets. The dietician will guide you about these. The British Diabetic Association also publishes a regular newspaper, *Balance*, which carries information about such foods, drinks and sweets. It also gives useful recipes, and you are recommended to join the Association and attend its local meetings.

Copies of the newspaper may even be available at your clinic and you could get one to read in the waiting room or on your way home. For information write to: The Secretary General, British Diabetic Association, 10 Queen Anne Street, London WIM OBD. If you decide against giving your child sweets at all, please let him have pocket money to spend on other things.

Once you have grasped the basic facts of diabetic care you may get a copy of the cookery book prepared for the British Diabetic Association by Pamela Robinson and Audrey Francis, *Successful Diabetic Cookery*. It may be on sale at your local BDA branch, possibly even at your diabetic clinic and certainly from the British Diabetic Association headquarters at the address given above. While it is by no means necessary it does extend your range of cooking and by providing some luxuries may reduce the temptation to eat cake and other sugary products.

Lastly, the British Diabetic Association publishes another *most* useful list of the branded or proprietary foods which are on sale at your usual grocer or supermarket. It contains the exchange value of each so that you can give your diabetic child the right amount of whatever the rest of the family is eating. It is known as "Calorie Countdown". It is most useful and is highly recommended. Again, it may be on sale at your local BDA branch or even at your clinic but if not you can get it from BDA headquarters at the above address. It reduces the anxiety and difficulty, especially for working mums who do not have enough time for special cooking. Diabetic children may be encouraged to visit the supermarket with a parent and the list. They can then identify the products on the shelves and discover the diabetic exchange values. By playing this game, possibly in a group from the clinic, the child becomes familiar with appropriate helpings of his favourite foods and independence is fostered.

Diets

There are, of course, other kinds of meal in which *all* articles of food are weighed and where a diet sheet is most carefully followed. They are as effective as the above method but are more difficult and less normal so that they have fewer followers. Other doctors have recommended a 'free diet' for all children, by which they mean that the child may eat what he wishes with the possible exception of sweets and cakes. This is a popular method where practised but we have not found it to be satisfactory, perhaps because of our unfortunate British preoccupation with eating large amounts of carbohydrate including sweets and biscuits at any time. The poorer results are generally apparent to the physicians and are likely to damage the child's health in the long run. There are rather uncommon exceptions when the physician will actually recommend such a free diet for special circumstances.

Normality again

The first principle in treating diabetic children is the assurance of a life as normal as any other. In relation to food this really means no more than spacing satisfactory meals at regular intervals during the day so that the energy flow can 'get through the doors' before the insulin effect is lost, the doors start closing and the energy (as glucose) builds up in the blood and is washed out in the urine. Mothers in our hospital soon notice, for example, that their child is fed from the same food trolley as everyone else and not from a special tray that marks him out as being different.

Having explained the Good Food System we should now emphasise that every child must have *enough* carbohydrate to meet his needs. If we do not give it to him, then even the saintliest child will succumb at times to temptation and will take more either at home or at the homes of friends or neighbours. Try to keep the carbohydrate as 'crude' as possible for reasons already given (p.10). Bran may be taken as Bran Flakes instead of Cornflakes and pure bran, inexpensively bought at your Whole Food shop can be added to soups, stews, etc. I make my own porridge with rolled oatmeal to which I add bran before cooking it — about 1 part of bran to 5 of oatmeal. Try getting the family onto wholemeal bread instead of nasty white plastic sliced bread. It is delicious when toasted.

Such 'crude' or whole food helps the diabetic to deal with carbohydrate. It takes the intestine rather longer to digest it (and that does *not* mean that it is indigestable) so that the glucose is more slowly released from the starch. It therefore gets into the bloodstream more slowly so that the glucose level is lower and the glucose slips more easily through the 'doors' which may be closing as the day progresses and the insulin effect is lost. Those who believe in the further slowing of starch digestion and glucose absorption by GUAR GUM may find products (e.g. crispbread) which contain it. It is not necessarily attractive but if it helps it is as sensible as increasing the insulin dose.

If the original number of exchanges leaves your child hungry for carbohydrate, then it is perfectly correct to give him more, provided you let your doctor and/or the clinic know. The doctor will then adjust your child's exchanges. For example, the diet mentioned above could be increased immediately to 23 exchanges by adding one to each meal and snack so that the list would now read 4, 3, 5, 3, 5, 3. At the same time or within a few days the insulin dose might need to be adjusted to deal with this.

Older children may enjoy shopping with you at your local supermarket and if you have time to spare may use the BDA's exchange list and proprietary food list to select what is most appropriate as well as economic.

WARNING: Although you may pick up useful tips from other parents of diabetic children, *never* make the mistake of thinking that their child's treatment or problems are the same as yours. You can be seriously upset and even misled if you do because every child's case is treated separately depending upon his diabetes, his parents, his home, his emotional stability, his age and so on.

If you have a question, then ask the doctor and not anyone else in the waiting room. The senior doctor has 'seen it all' whereas most mothers fortunately have no more than one affected child and may or may not, for all you know, be making a success of his care.

Advice service

Although the word 'diet' has been carefully avoided so as to stress the essential normality of the kind of meals your child should have, we are still very dependent on our dieticians who are trained in the scientific basis of good eating. Just as the British Diabetic Association dietician guides their publications, so your clinic may have a dietician who is very willing to discuss with you anything relating to your child's meals. She may also arrange cooking demonstrations at appropriate intervals, e.g. how to make your child's eating more exciting at Christmas-time or for a party. Please do not hesitate to ask for her as soon as you arrive at the clinic. Assuming that your hospital has one she will normally be present or at least available.

About sweetness and some sweetening agents

We would all be much healthier if we ate less sugar but unfortunately we do like sweet food and are comforted and bribed from infancy with sweets, chocolate and sweet fizzy or non-fizzy drinks. Not only our teeth but perhaps our hearts suffer and teenagers may become spottier in proportion to the amount of sugar taken in sweets and chocolate.

By the time children have become diabetic they are probably 'hooked' on sweetness and it may be too late to get them off it. Those who *can* do without sweets and sweet foods should do so but for those who *cannot* you should try substituting saccharin in one of a range of preparations available from the chemist. Alternatively you may add sorbitol or fructose to recipes. These contain as much energy as sugar and are therefore of no use to slimmers. It is not certain that they offer definite advantages to diabetics since the body simply converts them to glucose anyway. If an adult takes more than 60 grams daily of either, diarrhoea may result and they should not be taken as pure powders sprinkled on, for example, fruit.

I am not personally opposed to children, whose taste for sweets was developed before they became diabetic, having a very modest amount of confectionery. As with most things it is excess, intemperance, which is harmful. Total prohibition has a bad habit of causing backlash (e.g. alcohol prohibition in the U.S.A. in the past). When applied to a diabetic child whose parents have previously given him sweets, prohibition may lead to secret eating, bad conscience, parental suspicion, accusation, deteriorating relationships and defiance. If allowed 20 grams (2/3 ounce) per day, sweets could be distributed to follow meals and preferably about an hour after an insulin injection so that the glucose can be consumed. Special diabetic sweets are usually less exciting but can be used in rather greater quantity. There is also of course a dental argument against sweets (p.70) and happy is the child who prefers fruit, potato crisps or even dulse! Diabetic chewing gum has its supporters.

The carbohydrate exchange value of popular national confectionery will be found in the Calorie Countdown (see p.43). Popular sweet fizzy drinks contain a lot of sugar and should be avoided. Substitutes are available however. An excellent low-calorie (no sugar) range is marketed by both Boots and Schweppes while those made by Beechams (the Bitter Sweet range) contain some fructose but one full can is less than ½ an exchange. Sugar-free concentrated squashes are also available. Ice cream of course is permissible in amounts equivalent to one exchange (equivalent to a single plain ice as manufactured for example by Walls).

There is no reason why your child should not go to children's parties or picnics with others. Children often prefer savoury to carbohydrate foods on such occasions and you can probably estimate quite easily the amount of bread in the sandwiches. If you are in doubt you can make up a pack of food for the occasion and explain to the hostess that your child is diabetic and should eat his own things. The occasional unrestricted party however is unlikely to be harmful especially if you discuss with doctor or nurse how much extra soluble insulin might be taken to cope with any minor excess. With experience you can probably judge that for yourself.

Alternative diets

The BDA Carbohydrate Exchange List is not comprehensive. British families whose original communities were overseas in Africa or Asia may well follow traditional practices in the selection and preparation of food. Other families already living in overseas countries may wish to use this book for guidance. It cannot include detailed exchange lists for every community but each community may use its principles to prepare its own exchange list. Dieticians in Britain, in Africa and Asia have exchange lists which make this a simple exercise and you should seek their help. The Food and Agriculture Organisation of the United Nations provided in 1975 an updated annotated bibliography of food composition tables covering over 70 countries in every continent and providing much helpful advice. Most countries therefore have detailed food tables in their own language or are neighbours of countries with such tables and similar eating tastes.

The dietician needs only to list the common carbohydrates in your child's daily food, look them up in the tables and write down how many grams of each are equivalent to one 10 gram exchange. National diabetic associations, where such exist and are active, may already have done this and you should enquire of your doctor and or government health department.

5. EXERCISE

There is little more to say about exercise except to stress its importance as a method of keeping the blood glucose level as near normal as possible.

Our experience of diabetic adventure camps confirms this. Every year we find that young people come to camp on their usual doses of insulin. As soon as they get involved in climbing, sailing and canoeing (and especially if they fall into the water sometimes!) they pass less sugar in their urine and their insulin needs fall. Within a week and in spite of excellent meals their insulin doses may have been cut to ¾ or even ½. It helps of course to site our camps some miles from a tuck-shop and to provide only low calorie drinks!

Exercise need not be carried to the point of exhaustion. Indeed steady moderate exercise like walking, cycling and swimming may be best. Almost any sport is possible although most doctors advise diabetics to avoid rock-climbing and under-water swimming for reasons that will become obvious (see insulin reaction p.58). Football, rugby, hockey, lacrosse, tennis, golf (especially perhaps golf), basket ball, volley ball, gymnastics, athletics, swimming, riding, skating and skiing are all possible and indeed desirable.

Young diabetics should have company when they go walking far from help and should avoid swimming far out of their depth or on their own. In swimming pools it is wise to let the pond-master or swimming instructor know that he is a diabetic receiving insulin.

6. HOW DO WE KNOW TREATMENT IS CORRECT?

Our ideal objective is to keep the child diabetic's blood level between 3 and 8 mmol/1 (54 and 144 mg per 100 ml). The reasons will become clearer as you read on. Clearly we cannot know we are doing so unless we are regularly checking blood specimens through the day and every day and for most families that is still impracticable.

At its simplest we know he is not in any immediate danger if he is not excessively thirsty and is not passing urine often and in large volumes (p.   ).

We can however get an idea of blood level by checking the amount of glucose in his urine since it is washed out through the kidneys in increasing amounts when the blood level passes 10 mmol/1 (180 mg per 100 ml).

Testing urine samples

The diabetic child's urine should be tested regularly for glucose and ketones. Should he be doing the tests himself, the results should be confirmed by an adult. Cases of serious illness have occurred because young children misinterpreted the result of the test or recorded it wrongly either in error or because of fear that their parents may be cross or at least disappointed at a bad result.

With perfect control there should be no or only occasional

glucose in the urine and no ketones. The greater the amount of glucose, the more obvious it is that control is poor. Should ketones appear *as well as* glucose, then medical advice is required *without delay*. *Please remember* that children can pass into very dangerous coma (p.63) because parents fail to do or check this test. Ketones may appear in the absence of glucose and are then of much less importance and need no action.

Ketone testing

Your doctor will prescribe Acetest tablets or Ketostix strips but you are advised to test for ketones only on those days when the patient shows a + + + + result for glucose. Place a drop of his urine on a tablet or dip a Ketostix in the urine and judge its colour at 30 seconds with the chart provided.

Glucose testing

Your doctor will prescribe Clinitest apparatus. Holding the dropper absolutely straight up and down put 5 drops of urine and 10 drops of water into the little test-tube. Add one of the tablets. The mixture will bubble and the tube will become very hot. Wait for 15 seconds after the bubbling stops, shake the tube and compare the colour with the chart which comes with the tablets. Record the test as negative, tr, +, + +, + + + or + + + +. There are a number of catches to doing this test and one is that if there is too much glucose in the urine the colour may not develop properly. If there is reason to suspect the result, the test should be repeated using only 2 drops of urine and 13 drops of water. *Keep the tablets away from small children*. Should a child take one in mistake for a sweet it will boil in his mouth just as in the test-tube and, since it may stick to the surface of the mouth lining, it can produce hideous damage. Some clinics prefer a paper strip system such as keto-diastix. Here the strip is dipped into urine for 2 seconds, the excess is shaken off and the colour is

Table 1 Record of urine testing

Date	Dose of Insulin in units		Test				Ketones	Remarks
	Soluble	Isophane	1	2	3	4		
14/3	16	30	Tr	0	0	+	-	-
15/3	16	30	0	++	+	Tr	-	Mild hypo 7 a.m.
16/3	16	30	+	+++	0	Tr	Nil	-
17/3	16	30	Tr	0	0	Tr	-	-
Etc.								
Etc.								
Etc.								

compared with a chart. It is simple and convenient since it is as effective if it is simply passed through the urine stream for 2 seconds. This means it can be used easily when away from home or even out in the country since it does not require equipment. Parents should remember however with ketodiastix that a positive ketone test on the same strip (it indicates both glucose and ketones) is important only if there is $++++$ of glucose.

Urine testing should be done at recommended times. The usual times are:

1. On wakening. Pass urine and discard. Half an hour later pass urine again and test the specimen.* (The urine that has been in the bladder all night is not entirely satisfactory although the result can sometimes be helpful and your doctor may ask you to do it.)
2. Before lunch.
3. Before tea.
4. Before bed.

For specimens 2 and 3, the child should certainly have emptied his bladder at the mid-morning and mid-afternoon 'breaks' from classes, and for specimen 4 he should have emptied his bladder in the mid-evening.

Record these results in a book with hard covers. Line the pages as shown in Table 1.

It is a good idea to start this in hospital so that you can get the staff to help you with difficulties. *Please* add up the numbers of urine tests before you bring the child to the clinic. This saves the doctor's time and the time of those other parents and children in the waiting room. You need simply write on the page something like this: Total since last seen 141 tests, 80 negative, 20 traces, 15 $+$, 10$++$, 10 $+++$, 6 $++++$, or whatever the scores may have been.

Where a pre-lunch urine is difficult to obtain (school lunch etc), specimen 2 may be omitted except at weekends and on holidays.

---

* This double voiding may be impossible to adhere to in very young diabetics

Testing urine collections

Some clinics will, in addition to the above, or perhaps even instead of it, wish to check the amount of glucose lost by the child in 24 hours. This is done by saving ALL the urine passed in that time. The volume is then measured and the concentration of glucose in it is determined. The day's loss of glucose can then be calculated. It is important, of course, to note the starting time of the collection. Say it is 8 a.m. The child empties his bladder completely at 8 a.m. into the toilet and that is flushed away. From then up to and *including* 8 a.m. on the next day all urine is voided into a suitable bottle (the laboratory normally provides such) and the lot is sent for testing.

A variant of this test is to break the 24 hours into shorter periods, e.g. (a) 8 a.m. to noon; (b) noon to 4 p.m.; (c) 4 p.m. to 8 p.m.; and (d) 8 p.m. to 8 a.m. The glucose loss in each period can then be found and this may guide the physician as to the dose of which insulin (short or intermediate action) he should change in the morning and for evening. I have always been a little sceptical about the normality of a child's behaviour on such a day of urine collection. Where he is as active as usual and of course cooperative the system may be useful.

Colour vision

Do you know that some people cannot distinguish red and green? It is quite common and people whose jobs require them to see these colours (e.g. railway drivers) are tested before appointment. Other people cannot distinguish blue and yellow.

Now look at the range of colours in tests for urine glucose — blue, green, yellow, orange, brick! Parents and children doing urine tests need to have normal colour vision. We now test the colour vision of both parents and children at our diabetic clinic. It only takes a minute and does not involve clever answers to difficult questions. If you are in doubt about your colour vision or if other people think it is odd, why not ask to be tested. A friend of mine did not know he was colour blind until he bought a new car. His family thought its colour-scheme was dreadful. He thought it was an entirely different colour — grey.

Interpreting urine results

At first — and always if you feel uncertain yourself — you will want a doctor or a specially experienced nurse to interpret the test results and to guide your changes of insulin dose. You have nothing to worry about — they will always be willing to help. Whether the sample or the collection system just described are used, the glucose loss at certain periods in the 24 hour day is viewed against the effects on the known carbohydrate intake of the selected insulins given once or twice a day. Look back at p.21 to get the average duration of activity of short-, intermediate- and long-lasting insulins. Let us imagine a child who is having short and, intermediate insulins such as soluble and isophane. Then:

1. Heavy glucose loss in sample 2 or in collection A may indicate a need to increase the morning injection of soluble insulin.
2. Little or no glucose loss in sample 2 or collection A but heavy loss in sample 3 or collection B may point a need to increase the intermediate (e.g. isophane) dose in the morning.
3. Heavy loss in sample 4 with none in next morning's sample 1 or heavy loss in collection C but little in collection D suggests that the evening injection of soluble insulin is inadequate but that the child is having enough inter-mediate insulin.

Decisions are not always so easily made and you will often want medical and nursing help in your early weeks. There will be day to day variation in results. That shouldn't surprise us in a country where children may be outside and highly active in the sun one day but sitting watching television or painting pictures next day indoors as the rain pours down.

Quite apart from the value of urine samples in guiding the doses of insulin, the results of testing do indicate (where correctly tested and honestly recorded) the standard of control. When the results are added up for a period of 1 to 2 months I accept as reasonably satisfactory:

At least half of the tests — Negative

2/3 of the tests + or less

Not more than 1/5 + + + +.

Blood glucose level

Almost anyone can get a good idea of the blood level of glucose by using one of the chemical strips. Dextrostix has been the most commonly used one. The pulpy end of a warm finger is pricked in a way demonstrated to you by your doctor and a drop of blood is transferred to the chemical paper. It is allowed to act on it for one minute and it is then washed off with a gentle stream of cold water. The colour of the paper when compared with a chart indicates the glucose level. In the past it has been enough to know if it is too low (p.58) or too high (p.62). Now, however, the coloured end can be pressed dry in a paper tissue and the depth of colour measured more accurately in an electronic monitor of which several effective British models are available. I use the Hypocount made by the Hypoguard company (p.29) but there is little to choose between them. They are not available free to diabetics on the N.H.S. but some hospital clinics have a few to lend out for special purposes. However, the price is not prohibitive and as sales increase it may fall as in the pocket calculator market.

Such monitors were popularised in 1979 by the belief that the long-term complications of diabetes may be avoidable if the blood glucose level is held within normal limits most of the time. Diabetics have been buying them for their personal use (about £70 to 80 in early 1980) and parents have bought them so that they may more accurately supervise their diabetic child's treatment. I have one 9 year-old who happily checks not only her own blood glucose but that of her play-mates and any baby-sitter too old or too benign to offer resistance.

A new chemical strip (BM-Test-Glycemie 20−800 by Boehringer) is now available and the manufacturer claims for it several advantages — it makes possible estimation of blood glucose values between 20 and 800 mg per 100 ml (1.1 to 44.0 mmol/1), it does not need an electronic monitor, it does not involve a washing and drying stage and the colour does not fade. You can therefore take it to your doctor or clinic and have it checked. Trials reported in May 1980 suggest that such strips may make monitors unnecessary. Unfortunately your doctor cannot prescribe either Dextrostix or the BM Test free on the N.H.S. at present. They are issued for selected patients by hospitals but can be bought privately although not inexpensively.

The blood glucose level is usually determined routinely at diabetic clinic visits. Your doctor would like it to be less than 10 mmol/1 (180 mg per 100 ml) even one hour after a meal. He will certainly take the time of the last meal into consideration when he interprets the result and adjusts the insulin doses.

HbAl$_c$

HbAl$_c$ is part of the pigment that accounts for the red colour of blood. It has been studied intensively recently since it is claimed to give a good indication of the standard of diabetic control over the previous *weeks* rather than hours. It is valuable therefore in detecting those patients whose recorded urinary control is fictional or semi-fictional and especially those who ensure good control only for clinic visits! On the other hand, it is reassuring if a patient's control is poor at a clinic visit since it may show that overall control has been good. It is now widely used but may not yet have been completely evaluated.

57

7 SHORT-TERM COMPLICATIONS

Before you take your newly diabetic child home you should be familiar with some important complications which may occur immediately. All of them are easily recognised.

Disturbed eye-sight

Diabetes can cause serious harm to eye-sight in the long-term (p.72) but you should remember that, if your child was admitted to hospital very ill and in need of intra-venous therapy, it may take a few weeks for his vision to recover its sharpness. This is probably due to watery changes which the eye will correct completely for itself in a few weeks. So don't worry and don't rush off to have his eyes tested.

Insulin reactions

Insulin reactions are better named hypoglycaemic reactions or simply hypoglycaemia. This long word means that the level of glucose is too low (below 2.2 mmol/1 or 40 mg per 100 ml). As the level falls, the body tries to push it up again since the brain needs a good supply. In order to do this the boy's other glands begin to produce chemicals (we call these special chemicals hormones) which oppose insulin and release glucose from stores into the blood. The funny feelings the child experiences and his appearance are caused by these hormones. If they fail to release enough glucose in time the brain behaves a little like the brain affected by alcohol but it can be so upset by lack of glucose that a convulsion occurs. Hypoglycaemia always develops quickly and this distinguishes it from the much more dangerous ketoacidosis (too many ketones in the blood). Remember please that hypoglycaemia is rarely dangerous even if it looks rather alarming. A primary school teacher in Edinburgh put them in perspective when she described them as 'wee turns'. Even unconsciousness and convulsions are easily treated in time to prevent any lasting damage. All children in our hospital are given an insulin reaction on the day before discharge and in the presence of their parents. The child then knows what it feels like and the parents know what it looks like. The reaction is then ended by the parents giving the child glucose. The child and parents then experience together the rapid recovery to normal.

Symptoms

The following symptoms indicate varying degrees of severity.

Mild: Feels hungry, dizzy or faint.
Looks pale or flushed.
Skin moist or clammy.
Tremor particularly of the hands.

Moderate: Emotional and not thinking clearly.
Unsteady on feet.
Heart may be felt beating rapidly.
Eyes wandering or squinting.

Severe: Slumps or falls.
Resists help.
Very confused and may cry out.
Loses consciousness.
Convulses.

Each child behaves a little differently under such conditions and you will quickly recognise the early signs in your youngster's case. When there is too little glucose in the blood there will be none to enter the urine. Urine testing will therefore give a blue colour (negative). Note that the urine test may be misleading, for the urine in the child's bladder may have been there for some hours and, if some of it collected there at a time when there was too much glucose in the blood, it will contain glucose. On the other hand, a fresh specimen, if it can be obtained, will contain no glucose.

Causes

Insulin reactions may be caused by having too little food after an insulin injection (e.g. a stomach upset, a bad mood — 'I won't eat that', too long to wait for a meal, the sudden burning up of energy in an energetic game near to meal-time, chilling in air or water particularly if wet).

When a child shows unmistakable signs of an insulin reaction he should be given glucose irrespective of what the urine shows. Insulin reactions (short of coma) are quite common and are easily treated.

Precautions

1. The child should wear an identity disc; pet shops make them cheaply and some clinics provide them. They are very much better than any kind of medical card to be carried in clothing because children almost always lose these. The name, address and telephone number should be engraved on one side of the disc and on the other the word DIABETIC. Should he ever become confused or even unconscious when away from home this would speed up the process of treatment and of contacting you.

There are commercially-available information systems which are rather nicer than doggy discs. They are:
Medic-Alert of 9 Hanover Street, London WIR 9HF. This service provides a rather superior bracelet which carries a London telephone number. In return for a fee, Medic-Alert hold particulars of the child in their record system. In an

emergency, the hospital to which he has been taken calls that number and is told the diagnosis and the action to be taken. It needs to be kept up to date.

SOS Talisman is a very useful device designed rather like a watchcase and it is available in chrome or gold as a pendant or, with shoulders, for adding to a watch-strap. When unscrewed it reveals a folded strip of card on which is written extensive medical information. This is grouped under 3 headings in 3 European languages so that it may be easily examined in any part of Europe or indeed in most places your child is likely to visit. You can easily update it. It is readily available at good watchmakers and jewellers.

Medi-gen is a tube not unlike those worn by domestic pets on their collars but adapted for medical purposes and marked with a red cross. The information is rolled into a tube and carried inside it. Again the information is easily updated. You may find it locally available or you may write for information to A. L. Simpkin and Co. Ltd., Market Division, Hunter Road, Sheffield.

2. It is unwise to allow a diabetic child to go off walking or cycling alone for long distances or to swim unaccompanied, but then company is normal at this age.

3. Avoid long delays between meals. Be regular and prompt and encourage him to be so too.

4. The child should always carry a little box with some tablets of glucose in it (obtainable at any chemist). Glucose is preferred to sugar or sweets. Sometimes the school teacher will keep some in his or her desk for use in emergencies only. While useful for treatment glucose may be less satisfactory than 'crude' carbohydrate (e.g. wholemeal bread) in the prevention of attacks.

Treatment (see symptoms, p.59)

If he is only *mildly* affected start his meal immediately or at least give him a biscuit or a sweet, e.g. barley sugar and follow that with his meal as soon as possible.

If he is *moderately* affected make a solution of sugar or glucose 3 teaspoonfuls to a cup of water or squash. Help the child to take it in small sips. It is sometimes necessary to let it trickle between his teeth.

If he is *severely* affected then, if your doctor has given you a supply of *glucagon* to keep at home, inject it into him as described below. If you do not have glucagon then send for your doctor or an ambulance. Until they arrive try to trickle a little glucose into his mouth and if he is unconscious lay him semi-prone i.e. flat and half-turned into the prone position with his head on one side. *Keep calm*. He will be all right.

Glucagon is a powerful safe hormone which helps to release glucose from store so that the blood level rises. In our clinic we ensure that all our diabetic children have two packets of it at home. Parents keep an eye on the expiry date and ensure that unused glucagon is replaced before it is time-expired. Make sure you know how to prepare the glucagon quickly. This is very easy. Then inject all of the glucagon solution into a muscle. I prefer the upper and outer part of the buttock and we supply parents with long sterile needles so that they can inject the solution deeply. A comatose child commonly starts to stir in about 10 minutes. He must then be given glucose by mouth followed by something to eat since otherwise the blood glucose may fall again.

Diabetic ketoacidosis

This is the really dangerous complication of childhood diabetes. Your child is likelier than not to have been in more or less severe ketoacidosis when first diagnosed. If it is not treated with insulin then the child will die — and yet a child known to be diabetic should never get seriously into his this problem ever again. It can always be recognised early and treated easily.

Symptoms

The child may or may not have an infection or stomach upset.

He becomes thirsty and passes large volumes of urine. This water loss causes rapid loss of weight. He may complain of severe abdominal pain. His eyes look sunken and his tongue becomes dry. His breathing becomes deep and gradually increases in rate ('air hunger'). The sweet smell of ketones can be detected in his breath (p.1) and vomiting is common. He becomes drowsy and eventually comatose.

This takes a day or more, perhaps 2 or 3 days to develop, During this time his urine will contain $+ + + +$ glucose on each occasion. It will be positive for ketones. Parents and children therefore should *always* test the urine for ketones (p.51) when there is glucose $+ + + +$. Should ketones be present and should they persist until the next specimen 3 hours later — *seek advice immediately*. This is particularly urgent if he is also vomiting.

Causes

Ketoacidosis is always due to lack of insulin. Apart from the first onset of diabetes the likeliest cause of ketoacidosis is infection. Infection seems to increase the need for insulin. Much less commonly, it is due to a failure to give insulin. This has been used by older disturbed children as a means of getting into hospital as an escape from home or school.

Precautions

Be aware of your child's normal fluid needs and frequency of passing water. If he becomes very thirsty and is passing much urine then *do please* check it for glucose and ketones even if he recorded it previously as negative for both. Ketoacidosis is not a complication to be played with. It is very dangerous but severe illness and death are quite unnecessary.

It is particularly important that camp and cruise leaders and others should be aware of his diabetes and of the urgent nature of treatment necessary for its correction.

Treatment

This book began with a description of this treatment. It can be carried out simply and effectively at home by a good doctor but if he is vomiting he *must* be in hospital.

'Hypo' verses 'ketoacidosis'

The main difference between these two complications lies in the speed of their development. A diabetic child who was well at 11 a.m. and is unconscious at 11.30 a.m. is probably hypoglycaemic.

A drowsy or comatose diabetic child who has been ailing over 24 hours with thirst, increased urination and vomiting is almost certainly in ketoacidosis. Of the two the latter is the more dangerous but it need never be severe if urine testing is conscientiously done and insulin correction is started early. A common error is to with hold the morning insulin from a child who wakes up ill with no appetite, with vomiting and with glucose $++++$ and ketones in the urine. They are almost always in urgent need of soluble insulin even although they are not eating or not keeping down food or drink. Be sure to get advice quickly. Delay is dangerous. If your doctor is unavailable, take the child straight to your clinic by car or ambulance.

'Somogyi- ing'

A Dr Somogyi (pronounced Saw-maw-ji) drew attention in 1959 to a rather paradoxical situation concerning urine tests and hypoglycaemia. He pointed out that a diabetic child could sometimes have a hypoglycaemic reaction but have a lot of glucose in his urine. Not only that but his urine record in each 24 hours could show remarkable swings from being free of glucose to containing $++++$.

He suggested that, if a child became hypoglycaemic, he could switch on other glands, the chemicals of which actually raise the blood glucose level. These glands could rather over-react so that the child's blood glucose would go too high and would spill into the urine. If the insulin were then increased again it would cause further hypoglycaemia and the glands would once more over-react to push the blood glucose up so that the urine would again contain excess. This see-saw behaviour does occur and may lead your doctor to cut the insulin dose in an attempt to stabilise the blood glucose level.

A glucose profile

Your clinic may suggest a 24-hour admission to prove or disprove what is often known as 'somogyi-ing'. The child is allowed to move freely around the investigation area. A fine tube is slipped through a puncture into a vein, where it remains quite painlessly. Small samples of blood are drawn from it during the day and night without disturbing the patient and without the blood loss being significant. Analysis of their glucose content enables adjustments to be made to insulin doses.

8. GOING HOME

As soon as your child is up and about in his hospital room and you know about insulin injections, simple but good meals, urine testing and how to recognise hypoglycaemia, you will be able to take him home. This will usually be about one week after admission. His urine may still contain glucose at this time because it is difficult to get normal exercise in hospital and the doctor may prefer to keep his blood glucose a little high so that the change of activity and of outside temperature at home will not precipitate hypoglycaemia.

Check list

In our unit the staff use a check list which is ticked off as each point is covered in preparation for discharge home. Perhaps you would like to go through it. Not all of it may be relevant, of course, in your community.

1. Good Food System explained
2. B.D.A. 'Carbohydrate Exchange List' supplied
3. Diabetic food weighing scales obtained
4. Diabetic cookery book
5. Calorie Countdown seen
6. Colour vision tested — child, mother, father
7. Urine test instruction complete — glucose; ketones
8. Testing agents supplied — glucose; ketones
9. Urine test result book prepared
10. Insulin(s) supplied
11. Insulin syringes (BS 1619 glass) supplied
12. Insulin needles supplied

13. Syringe sterilisation demonstrated
14. Spirit-proof case (Hypoguard) supplied
15. Spirit obtained
16. Insulin injector demonstrated: supplied
17. Insulin reaction demonstrated; treated
18. Glucagon supplied
19. Long needles for glucagon supplied
20. Identity disc/pendant/bracelet obtained
21. Introduction to Home Care Team
22. Family doctor informed of planned discharge date
23. Address of British Diabetic Association obtained
24. School Health Service informed by Hospital
25. 'Young Diabetics' leaflet supplied for parents

Home care team

If your clinic has a home care team, the nursing officer may have already made an appointment to call on you at home the day after discharge. Should there be matters that you do not yet understand or should you have personal or family matters which you fear might make diabetic care difficult, you will find her a good listener and friend who will respect your confidences.

School

Your child's school should certainly be told that he has developed diabetes since he needs his lunch punctually, may need to have a snack in class and should have teachers who can recognise and treat hypoglycaemia. A very few parents are secretive about their child's diabetes and insist that neither the school's doctor nor the teachers be told. While I can understand why they do so, I am quite clear that sharing this information with school's staff is very much to the child's advantage. The Scottish Health Education Unit at 21 Lansdowne Crescent, Edinburgh EH12 5EH produces a simple and attractive leaflet for school teachers. It is readily available to clinics and schools with the intention of placing a copy not only with the form teacher but *with each teacher* whom the child has (including P.E. and swimming) and it should be given out to new teachers each year. It is useful to the leaders of youth organisations and others involved for example with camps. The content is reproduced in Appendix 1 with the permission of the S.H.E.U.

9. THE CRYSTAL BALL

Predicting the future was probably already an old skill when King Saul consulted the Witch of Endor (1st Samuel chapter 28). History is full of witches and astrologers, prophets and gypsies who with or without financial incentive consulted their stars, cards, cauldrons or crystal balls and told their client's future. Shepherds and sailors developed necessary expertise in looking at the hills, the skies, the birds and berries for an indication of the coming weather. Those afflicted with rheumatism may know what tomorrow will be like by pain in their joints. Science now uses satellites. Doctors, of course, are deeply involved in what has become a science and so are the actuaries who decide how much your life insurance premium is going to be when you want a building society loan (or your diabetic child wants one in a few years time). They have calculated for cigarette smokers the risks of getting lung cancer or heart attacks and for the predisposition of other groups developing serious health problems at different ages as a result of influences which could be avoided. Childhood diabetes is one such disorder in which future complications can be very serious but *are preventable*. If doctors believed that they were still unavoidable and inevitable they would remain silent about them since the information could cause only anxiety to their parents.

The complications now to be described are probably preventable to a considerable extent by the best possible normalisation of the blood glucose level and other chemical processes which depend on it throughout life. This involves

69

careful attention to insulin injections (the nearer the patient gets to having insulin as if it were coming from a normal pancreas the better), to the use of Good Food and to taking sensible exercise. Parents who can instil into their child's mind such practices without causing boredom, frustration and rebellion will provide a great start to a normal life self-controlled by tolerable discipline. A happy trusting relationship in the years before getting diabetes is almost essential to success. On the other hand parents who fail at some point in their child's development to achieve co-operation and good control should remember that the development of severe complications requires poor control and that temporary rebellion in childhood or in adolescence still leaves years in which their child can establish a high standard of self-care. They should also remember that medicine has advanced very quickly in the past 20 years and that automatic computerised control of diabetes may be a fact within the next 20. It usually takes about 20 years before unsatisfactory control produces visible complications likely to impair seriously the quality of life.

Dental decay

It has been said that diabetic children are more susceptible to dental decay than others — or that the soft tissues of the gums are likelier to become infected. They may even have greater tartar formation. It is a little difficult to be sure of this in a country where children's teeth are very commonly decayed by sweets and poor prevention.

Everyone knows now that sugar has got a lot to do with dental decay. It acidifies the film which forms on the teeth (called plaque by dentists) and this eats away the enamel. If a diabetic child has excessive sugar in his mouth his teeth may be under prolonged attack but on the other hand if his blood glucose is normal and if he is eating crude carbohydrate (p.10) his teeth should be healthier provided that he brushes them correctly after meals.

Some doctors recommend that the young diabetic child should be wakened at 9-10 p.m. and given a snack of milk and biscuits to prevent hypoglycaemia overnight. If this is done the child's teeth should be brushed afterward since there is no practice more likely to rot teeth than to leave a child with mushy biscuit stuck to his teeth overnight. Apple and pear have had their advocates as a way to give a snack and to clean the teeth at night but some criticise their own fruity acidity as possibly harmful. Banana is claimed to be better while both cheese and nuts are quite effective. A child should never however eat nuts when sleepy or about to go to sleep in case he inhales one.

If sweets are allowed at all then chocolate is less harmful to teeth than are toffees, boilings or mints — and a quick crunch is much less harmful than sucking or letting a sweet disolve in the mouth gradually.

If the diabetic child should grow up in an area fortunate to have adequate fluoride in its water supply then of course his teeth will be more able to resist decay. Some dental clinics do take trouble to paint the teeth of diabetic children with fluoride. There may be some merit for diabetics in having fluoride mouth washes, using fluoride tooth paste or (probably best) allowing a small fluoride tablet to disolve very slowly in the mouth — perhaps overnight.

Fat loss and lumps

Since the earliest years of treating children with insulin a high proportion have developed changes at the sites of insulin injections. In some children the fat underneath the injection site begins to disappear so that, without breaking the skin at all, a rather unsightly hollow develops. In others — or even sometimes in the same child — fat accumulates at one or more injection sites and can produce a swelling like a half tennis-ball under the skin. It seldom worries boys but girls naturally do not like it. This complication may be inescapable in some diabetics but there is a feeling that it is commoner in children who always inject in exactly the same place. It is important therefore to develop a routine of moving the injection site daily (p.33) and of using not only the legs but the arms, the buttocks and the fat over the front of the abdomen (Fig. 6).

Affected areas take a long time (years perhaps) to return to normal if they are no longer used for injections. There is reason to believe that a change to highly purified pork insulins permits faster recovery especially perhaps if they are injected under the skin around the margins of a hollow.

Disordered growth

Poor control in childhood may significantly stunt growth because, although the necessary food for growing is being eaten, the absorbed building energy cannot be used (inadequate insulin) and is being lost through the kidneys in urine. It was commoner 20 years ago and may have been due in part to unnecessary strict diets.

If he is young enough when good control is again achieved, he may well be able to catch up to some extent. Even if he does not, short stature is a minor disability and does not threaten life.

Educational failure

While poor control does not by itself affect intelligence, it may interfere with education through hospitalisation, severe infections, hypoglycaemia and refusal to go to school. Poor school achievement leads to having a less skilled job than might have been possible otherwise — and less skilled jobs may make the achievement of good control that much more difficult.

Visual handicap

This is perhaps the most emotive subject in diabetes and I

would gloss over it if there were not now a growing belief that the best possible control of the blood glucose can indefinitely delay or prevent it. Retinopathy is a change in the tiny blood vessels of the 'movie camera' at the back of the eye known as the retina. It becomes visible to the physician in some cases after 20 years and develops further at varying pace. While it can be treated nowadays by laser beam (photocoagulation) it is depressing to know that diabetes still stands at the top of the causes of blindness in middle age in Britain. It is impossible for a child to think realistically in terms of 20 to 30 years ahead of him when he has a box of chocolates in front of him and it would be wrong to threaten him with this danger. Wise parents, however, will find their own ways of motivating him to cooperate as fully as possible with good diabetic control from an early age. It should be added, of course, that this kind of visual handicap is not associated with external changes in the eyes. They look perfectly normal. The patient can see no change when he looks at his eyes in a mirror. Nor will his family notice. Only the skilled physician looking through the pupil with his ophthalmoscope sees what is happening. Some research workers believe that even when early changes are visible they may be reversed (improved) by very strict diabetic control. If true, this is good news but how much better it is to prevent the changes ever happening. There are now methods, some chemical and some microscopical, by which physicians can watch the early development of change. They are difficult, however, and are not for general application.

In the earlier days of insulin treatment, diabetic children sometimes developed cataract (clouding of the lens of the eye) but improved treatment over the years has been associated with its disappearance. I have not found a single case in the 25 years of holding a large clinic.

Kidney failure

The blood vessel changes are not confined to the eyes. Similar changes in the kidneys lead to poorer function in the excretion of poisons and to loss from the blood of important protein. This damage takes place at about the same pace as that in the eyes although one process may be more obvious than the other. While the changes cannot, as in the eyes, be inspected by direct vision, they can be suspected by laboratory tests of the urine and proved by taking very tiny samples of the kidney using a special needle inserted into it during local or general anaesthesia.

Diabetic kidney can badly disable the patient and indeed shorten his life. While kidneys, unlike eyes, can at least be transplanted there are factors which make it rather more difficult in diabetics. Again — how much better to take care of the diabetes over the years and to prevent damage. Adult diabetic women are likelier to have urinary tract infections than are non-diabetics: the sugar in the urine attracting the germs. This may in turn lead to severe kidney damage or failure. Diabetic children who are well cared for and clean are not in my experience any likelier to get kidney infections than their non-diabetic friends.

Nerve damage

You probably know already that the feet of elderly diabetics are given special attention since there is a likelihood of damage and infection leading to serious changes — even gangrene. They are advised for example not to cut their own toe-nails and they are given advice about foot hygiene and the fitting of shoes. This is because the nerves carrying sensation from the feet become less efficient in elderly diabetics and as a result they do not feel cuts, abrasions and infections. When this happens in the elderly whose blood supply may already be impaired it can lead to amputation.

The diabetic child, however, is unaffected by this problem although, again, poor control over many years may render him susceptible in time.

Heart disease

Diabetics are prone to develop disease of arteries and those which supply the heart muscle may become narrowed with age. There is still uncertainty as to why the *non*-diabetics get coronary artery disease. As mentioned before (p. 38) the excessive intake of animal fat or of sugar have been suspected and smoking undoubtedly plays a big part. It has also been claimed that replacing animal fats with some vegetable fats (e.g. corn oil or sunflower oil) may actually protect the arteries from being silted up, as it were, and narrowed. What is quite clear is that being fat, smoking and taking too little exercise are harmful to the non-diabetic. It is very likely therefore that they are harmful to diabetics and the advice given in this book is directed toward prevention.

Pregnancy problems

Girls whose diabetes has been well controlled really have very little trouble in pregnancy provided that they receive proper attention at that time. Those, however, whose diabetic care has been poor since childhood; while at no risk of dying in pregnancy, may suffer rapidly increasing damage to vision or the loss of the child. It should be emphasised that there have been great improvements in diabetic care during pregnancy in recent years.

10. GAMES DIABETIC CHILDREN PLAY

Parents who themselves enjoyed a healthy happy childhood and even parents who became diabetic in adult life may find it difficult to identify with a child whose life has been abruptly affected by such an experience.

Injections may be an ordeal at first to very young or very sensitive children but they are soon tolerated as a routine by most (a visit to diabetic camp to see 50 others cheerfully injecting themselves is a helpful experience — see p.86). What bothers the otherwise normal diabetic child in an otherwise normal home is any curtailment of freedom which makes him different from his friends — picked out and set apart. In a community in which sucrose has been the ultimate reward from infancy it may be its prohibition that leaves him deprived and an outcast from his social group homing in on the local tuck shop. Many will fall to temptation whether deprived of pocket money or not and there are always friends and relatives who will provide the forbidden food.

An excursion into secret eating of sweets and cakes or of drinking sugary pop leads, if it is even a little bit excessive, to glucose in the urine and to the asking of questions, the challenging of answers, accusation and perhaps punishment (e.g. no pocket money) in an attempt to prevent its happening again.

False recording

The simplest attempt to escape a confrontation with parent

and doctor is simply to report the urine test as O (negative) instead of $+ + + +$. Such an action is almost always apparent to the doctor and is usually spotted at the next clinic visit since the clues are obvious. There are of course many occasions when the doctor realises that the *parent* has entered the false record, little effort having been made to achieve control, so that a perfect record book seems the obvious way to escape an otherwise embarrassing interview.

'Fiddling' the urine test

The 'fiddled' test is only a more sophisticated form of falsely recording the results. The test is seen to be performed, the result is agreed and another 'con trick' is recorded! The simplest form is to test someone else's normal urine — a brother's or a sister's perhaps.

Others dilute the urine in the toilet with water so that a very sugary specimen becomes a + or a trace. One young lady carried out the test in the kitchen with her mother watching her for weeks — placing 5 drops of water in the test tube followed by 10 drops of water and the Clinitest tablet! No urine was used in the test at all! An even more resourceful boy was accompanied to the toilet by his suspicious mother. With his back turned he passed urine into a container for testing and handed it back to her. She thought his action somewhat unusual and found that he actually had a small bottle of water inside his trousers with which to dilute the specimen even in her presence!

Where children go to such lengths the educational programme is failing or relationships are wrong and need help. It is for this reason that I believe that the child previously hooked on confectionery is better to have a known moderate amount of it adequately covered with insulin than an unknown amount secretly eaten at unpredictable times without an appropriate insulin dose to take care of it.

There is of course another group of children whose abuse of their diabetes is a protest — a defiant contravention of rules imposed by 'them', the normal world of adult authority. They are a difficult group — usually hurt in some way before they became diabetic. Too often they have good reason to protest. Life has treated them unkindly or it has overindulged them without loving constraint. Even those adults who try to help them are subjected to their anger and bitterness. They 'don't care' and feel compelled to strike out at the society which hurt them. They can be helped but it is slow, commonly sad, and often thankless work.

Refusing meals

The refusal to eat breakfast after having had the morning insulin dose is a powerful weapon. It may be as naked as that — 'so now what are you going to do?' At other times there is the more subtle complaint of 'feeling ill' and being unable to eat. It is commoner in the very young who can usually be saved from the error of their ways by giving their morning carbohydrate exchanges as a drink. Older children who do this need help and often respond well to a period of assured love and attention (p.83).

Omitting insulin

Very occasionally I have dealt with sad cases where children have failed to give themselves insulin (and an uncaring family has not noticed) or have pretended to give themselves insulin but have misdirected it onto the carpet. Such children have wanted to escape from an unhappy situation to a familiar and acceptable hospital one and have required considerable help over a long period to adjust and become independent.

Do please keep your insulin safely. Small supplies are safer than big ones and it is simple to note how long a single container of 10 ml normally lasts your child. By taking care in this way you can help prevent the serious accidents when too little (or too much) is taken.

Pretending hypoglycaemia

Some children occasionally feign hypoglycaemia in order to avoid something they do not want to do or somewhere they do not want to go. The fact that their urine contains glucose (even + + + + does not exclude hypoglycaemia since it only tells us that the blood glucose has been high since the bladder was previously emptied. The simplest way to determine the truth is to do a blood test (p.56). This will show you whether the blood glucose is truly low. If you are having this kind of problem your doctor will probably give you a supply of a paper strip such as Dextrostix with instruction how to use it.

11. MAKE YOUR CHOICE

You *must* read the previous sections before you read this one. Since you now know that serious complications are believed to be preventable or at least reduced in severity by keeping the amount of glucose in the blood normal for as much of each 24 hours as possible, it is for you to achieve this. When you go on holiday you can decide whether you will travel 1st or 2nd class on the train or ship, or 1st or Economy class on the aircraft. When you stop overnight on tour you usually have a choice of Bed and Breakfast or of hotels allotted stars in proportion to their excellence. Diabetics do not, in the British health care system, need to pay more money to get the best care *but* they can choose how hard they will try to provide the best care for themselves. Young diabetic children are entirely dependent, of course, on the help of their parents or guardians — so you have a choice to make. The doctor/nurse team do not make the choice. Choice is the privilege of the parent or the youngster himself. The doctor/nurse team want young diabetics to have the best care and will give all the help they can.

Now look at the choice —

Stars	Description of control
O	Survival in serious doubt. No care. No tests or falsely reported tests. Perhaps no insulin or only irregular insulin (see Diabetic Hostels p.83).
★	Survival — with risks. Ignorance or rebellion. Few

tests or falsely reported tests. Eating anything at any time. Poor use of insulin. Thirst, large volumes of urine, ketonuria (ketones in the urine) and weight loss used as indication for visit to the doctor.

★★ Satisfactory diabetic future. Serious effort to get good control. Regular urine tests correctly reported. Urine tested for ketones whenever glucose 2 per cent (++++) present. Insulin injections given well at a rotation of sites. Dose adjusted to get good control. Good control defined as follows during each month:

More than half urine glucose tests NEG; ⅔ of all tests + (½ per cent) or less; not more than 1 in 5 of all tests ++++
and/or

a result judged satisfactory by the doctor on the basis of the *daily* loss of glucose in the urine. Mild hypoglycaemia quite common but hypoglycaemic coma (unconsciousness) quite uncommon.

★★★ Blood glucose kept in the normal range most of the time — intermittent insulin injections used along with blood glucose monitoring.

★★★-
★ Blood glucose kept in the normal range almost all the time — continuous insulin delivered by syringe-pump along with blood glucose monitoring.

★★★-
★★ Blood glucose always normal — maintained by pancreas replacement.

In the present state of knowledge most good parents and co-operative children will aim for ★★. But ★★★ and ★★★★ are possible for intelligent, stable people who have the equipment. Unfortunately ★★★★★ is still for the future.

Remember that while there may be the most serious short-term (i.e. in a few days) consequences of stopping treatment, the kind of long-term complications described on pages 72—75 result from years of poor control. Parents need not be distressed by occasional periods of poor control or even by a year or two when the child's behaviour prevents good control.

A declaration of war between parents and child over the subject of control may do more harm in the long run than will the high glucose level itself. How? By rendering the child deaf to discussion and reason.

Should you be going through a bad spell in terms of diabetic control, keep cool and work quietly and patiently toward better times. The child, or more probably teenager, may well decide to try harder as he/she becomes more responsible. I use 'she' also in this context because girls do often get the message about control when they begin to think of its effect on later babies.

12. DIABETIC HOSTELS

There are times when diabetic control becomes so bad that a child's life becomes a series of hospital admissions connected by brief and often unhappy spells at home. As a result his education is badly interrupted and his future employment is prejudiced. He may become 'hospital-dependent' and the changing hospital staff become his shifting and remote family. The reasons for this vary and do not concern us here although social and psychological circumstances are clearly important.

A number of diabetic hostels have functioned in Britain for such very unfortunate children. They provide comfortable living accommodation and usually both medical and nursing supervision. The children go to the local schools where they attempt normal studies, normal recreation and are subject to normal discipline. The teachers benefit from such advice as is provided in the S.H.E.U. leaflet *Young Diabetics* (p.67)

The programme provided by such hostels should not be restricted to board, lodging and diabetic care. Barnardo's hostel 'Cruachan' in Edinburgh places great emphasis on the child's emotional state, his home situation and on working toward reunion in more effective circumstances. Child Care staff are partnered by medical and nursing staff in providing a comprehensive service both in the hospital and in the child's home. The provision of Home Care Teams of child-orientated (paediatric) staff certainly helps reduce the demand for hostel vacancies and indeed for hospital beds for diabetic purposes.

13. YOUR GOOD HEALTH!

The correct use of carbohydrate exchanges and insulin does not make a child healthy! It only makes him a normal complete child.

Protection from infection

He still needs care to protect him from infections by immunisation. We live in a decade when most of the population have forgotten the death and disability caused by whooping cough in the first half of this century. We have painful memories however of ill children who might have been spared this disease had they acquired even partial protection from a vaccine which carries a much smaller risk, than does the disease itself. Just imagine for a moment the problems of a diabetic child with whooping cough — the insulin must be given daily but his paroxysms of coughing cause him to vomit part or all of his meals. How would you calculate the number of exchanges then? And it lasts for weeks. So do accept as much protection as the National Health Service freely offers — including BCG (against TB) since in the old days when tuberculosis was common, it was even commoner among diabetics. It is still included in our immunisation programme although this may change.

The best general protection against infection is good diabetic control. Germs love sugar.

Teeth

I must repeat the need for good care of the teeth. Children and young people look so much nicer with healthy teeth of their own. They smell nicer too! Some close-ups are really very nasty.

Smoking

Please set your child a good example by not smoking. The statistics of how much of life a smoker puffs away with each cigarette are well publicised. Add that to the effects of diabetes. It is a very harmful practice and entirely unnecessary to being a real man or an attractive woman. Diabetic children should not smoke. See that they are aware of the positive advantages of not doing so.

Drugs and alcohol

At what age do they start experimenting with these in your area? Both are more readily prevented than stopped.

Exercise

Encourage a pattern of healthy exercise according to age — walking, jogging, formal training on the track, cycling and ball games. Swimming too (p.18). Join them if you can in their (and your!) younger years.

Weight

Be a weight-conscious family without over-doing it. Use the height and weight charts to keep in the normal range. This has many good effects.

14. CHILDREN'S CAMPS

Most children love to go to camp with their friends and the diabetic child is no exception. Once his diabetes has stabilised he may go camping, *if* the camp leaders (teachers or youth organisation leaders) know he is a diabetic, the kind of problems that may arise and how they should be treated. It is unfair not only to the diabetic child but to all the other campers and staff to withhold this information or to let him go with uninformed people. Hypoglycaemia (too little sugar in the blood), perhaps even coma, in a remote area (perhaps even on a mountain) can be a major problem and it spoils the outing for everyone. Hypoglycaemia, you will remember, can be caused by unusual exercise, delayed food or exposure to cold and wet. These are common hazards of the British camper.

The British Diabetic Association runs camps for children in different age groups right up to school-leaving. They range from living in permanent accommodation and playing gentler games to getting a tent up on a mountainside after a day's trek by moor and water. They teach children how to cope with tests, injections and complications but all in the safe company of suitable staff. They are then in a much better position to camp without such cover on future occasions. They can join more safely with their non-diabetic friends at school and youth camps.

Some parents feel strongly (and I sympathise with their view) that they want their child 'to get away from diabetes and other diabetics' for holidays. Some doctors, perhaps those of a more romantic nature, feel diabetic school children should not be brought together for camps lest they should fall in love and have children with an increased chance of becoming diabetic. Life is a matter of perspective. The advantages of diabetic camps far outweigh the disadvantages.

The B.D.A. is looking further afield now and is providing camps outside Britain with the cooperation of diabetic associations in other countries. Think about it. Perhaps you could even help if you have camping skills and develop a good grasp of diabetic care.

15. TRAVELLING

Air travel

Air travel does not by itself disturb diabetic control and arrangements made by a good airline are usually sufficient for flights within Europe. It is wise however to consider carefully the unscheduled delays nowadays (I spend a significant part of my life in the world's airports!) and the following advice is offered.

Food on short-haul holiday charter flights may consist of sandwiches, biscuits, sliced cake etc, and may be short of protein as well as heavy on carbohydrate. Parents should enquire about the meals well before departure and make such arrangements for their child as may be necessary — taking a meal with them in a cabin bag.

Please remember to take *syringes, needles, swabs, insulin, glucose and glucagon* in your cabin baggage for the journey. You certainly can't get into the aircraft's hold at 30 000 feet and airlines do not enjoy unnecessarily unloading a large aircraft at some unscheduled stop on the route! It is wise to divide your medical supplies among your cases as well as to have some in your cabin bag i.e. syringes and insulin in each, some glucagon in each etc. Temporary loss of a bag is far from rare — it may speed off to Malaysia or Manitoba instead of Majorca! While it is likely to turn up in a few days (my range is from 3 days to 6 weeks), the period without supplies can spoil the earlier part of your holiday. Not all holiday resorts have helpful pharmacies, working telephones or doctors who speak English. And by the way — do ask the British Diabetic

Association about medical insurance cover.

Of much greater importance is the common problem of delayed departure. Operational difficulty may cause passengers to wait many hours while industrial action (usually at holiday season, of course!) may lead to delays of a day or two in over-crowded buildings and overwhelmed catering services. In hot climates, especially when airports are badly developed and staffed, such waiting can be distressing even to normal people. It can be dangerous to young diabetics and especially when mother and children may be travelling alone to join father in a developing country. The time of day or night and the day of the week (Islamic and Israeli weekends are not those of Europe) may affect the service.

Parents are strongly advised therefore to allow for such delays and Appendix 3 suggests the kinds of packs which they might take as a precaution. Fluids are most important since they may be unavailable, unsuitable, unsafe or just extortionate in price. Carry some water and diabetic squash or cans of low-calorie drink if the security services will permit them in the cabin. In any case it is wise for all long-distance travellers to carry water-sterilising tablets (e.g. Sterotabs, Boots).

Within Europe and in North-South intercontinental travel the diabetic child's meal times on the aircraft are likely to approximate to those at home. If they are a little later than at home then he can temporise with 1 to 2 exchanges from his travel pack and deduct them from the airline meal which follows.

In East-West/West-East intercontinental travel the passenger passes through different time-zones. The clock is advanced as he flies East and put back as he flies West. In long journeys to North America (particularly to the West coast) or the Far East this leads to some irregularity of meals. Airlines do their best to space them but the child diabetics control may get moderately disturbed. Parents may avoid this problem by leaving their watches on British time and by serving their own packed meals to the child at the usual times, covered by insulin given at the usual times. This will also take care of delays on the ground en route and the child will sleep during his normal British sleep hours.

On arrival at the end of the flight parents should plan to have some exchanges and fluids left to supply his needs during the usual formalities of immigration, health and currency control, luggage collection and customs.* Once at their destination it is usually a simple matter within their own capabilities and experience to adjust the exchanges and insulin so that he slides with as little disturbance as possible into the local meal-times.

Alternatively, experienced parents will simply accept the airline's meal-times on board but will use several little doses of soluble insulin to cover each major intake and will omit the intermediate insulin. They should take low-calorie drinks however. Urine may be tested en route (I suggest Ketodiastix and not Clinitest and Acetest/Ketostix under such conditions). Blood can be checked with Dextrostix with or without a monitor or with BM Glycemie 20-800.

Train, bus, car and ship

Surface travel has both advantages and disadvantages. Time change is naturally very much slower and so much less manipulation of insulin, meal and sleep times is needed.

It is usually possible to check in advance as to the availability of a buffet car on British rail journeys of any significant duration. Their range of sales is rich in carbohydrate and parents of a diabetic child are advised to carry a packed meal with them. This view has been re-inforced by a lightning strike of buffet car staff virtually throughout British Rail on the day this is written, with due apology 'for the incon-

---

* This can take a long time. In 1980 it has taken me 1 hour in London Heathrow and 2 hours in a developing country.

venience caused to passengers'. This is of small consolation to diabetics.

Sea travel is now mostly short ferry crossings and reasonable provision is usually available in the self service cafeteria or dining room.

Car travel has the merit of permitting the family to stop and eat when and where it wishes but before embarking on long haul scheduled bus services or tours it is wise to check what stops are planned and what meals will be available. Some reserve rations (packets of potato crisps, plain biscuits, cheese, apples and low calorie drinks) may be carried.

The most important precaution to take on all surface travel is a supply of motion sickness prevention pills if there is the slightest doubt about the diabetic child's stability in such transport. If there is a history of motion sickness it is wise to give the necessary pill at least half an hour before departure. Persistent vomiting after injecting the day's insulin may cause hypoglycaemia.

16. THE FAMILY ABROAD

Travel over short distances involves little change in the way of life. Since men now travel far afield in rather different circumstances than they did before the Second World War, they may live in cultures very different from home. The father who is thinking of taking his wife and family with him should explore the services available to the diabetic child. Information about the nature, number and times of meals may be discussed with the child's home doctor so that guidance may be given about the times and likely doses of insulin. Factors like environmental temperature, air-conditioning, swimming pools and play areas should be considered since children can be tremendously active in warm sunny countries. Suitable schools with good water supplies and acceptable meals should be sought.

Enquiries about the suitability of local clinics and the experience of the physicians with childhood diabetes are wise. The supply of insulin, urine and blood test reagents etc should be assured.

Children tolerate such changes remarkably well and given a reasonable hospital service, diabetic children are as tough as any others. A mother going for the first time to join her Muslim husband in an Islamic country need not worry about the effects of starvation during daylight on the diabetic child in Ramadan since he will be excused the full rigours of this period — the Koran having made provision for that. Hindu society also observes fast days but they, too, will not submit a diabetic child to what he cannot bear.

In any country it is inadvisable to consult anyone but a medical graduate about a child's diabetes. Herbalists and others may prescribe concoctions with quite profound (harmful) effects on diabetic chemistry.

Here are some questions which you should ask yourself should you be worried about your child abroad.

1. *Poor health, and weight loss*
   a. Is the child excessively thirsty?
   b. Are there symptoms of other illness, e.g. a cough, fever, diarrhoea, pain on passing water, a skin rash or is there illness in other members of the family or among house servants?
   c. Must he rise at night to pass urine or to drink?
   d. How satisfactory are his urine tests?
   e. Is his urine tested as often as it ought to be?
   f. Is the urine record correct or might it have been wrongly reported?
   g. Are relationships good at home, at school and out-of-doors?
   h. Is he known to eat all his meals?
   i. Is vomiting expected?
   j. In an older child is there any reason to suspect experimentation with cigarettes, alcohol, glue-sniffing?

2. *For poor control*
   a. Is the insulin dose correct?
   b. Is the insulin within its expiry date and has it been kept cool?
   c. Is the insulin being given?
   d. Is the injection site being changed daily?
   e. Might the insulin dose need to be changed?
   f. Might morning and evening injections be needed?
   g. Is the correct amount of carbohydrate being taken at the right times?
   h. Is extra sugar being taken secretly as chocolate, sweets or drinks?

i.   Is hypoglycaemia being overcorrected with glucose?

j.   Are there symptoms to suggest an infection (established or developing)?

3. *Loss of consciousness**

a. Has he been well until this suddenly happened during the past half-hour? (hypoglycaemia)

b. If so does he respond to carefully given glucose by mouth or to a glucagon injection?

c. Has he been out of sorts all day and showing glucose + + + + and ketones in urine?

d. Can you smell ketones in his breath?

e. Is his breathing deep and fairly slow?

f. Has he abdominal pain and vomiting?

If the answer to c, d, e and f is yes, secure immediate help.

---

* Excluding of course suspicions of head injury, poisoning or acute infection.

17. A LAST WORD

A last word to mothers

Every good mother does her best for her family and you will naturally try hard to give your diabetic child the happiest possible future. This can involve some hard decisions, especially if you are also wage-earning and not only enjoying your work but making a significant contribution to the family's standard of living. I do not suggest that you should give up your job altogether but you and your husband should decide that one responsible, fully informed adult is at home to send the child off to school in the morning and to receive him when he returns at lunch and/or in the afternoon. I am not advocating a constant nagging presence to check that the child does not trespass against the simple food rules — but rather that he accepts as natural a harmonious partnership in seeking the best possible standard of care.

I would like you to do two other things. The first is that you involve your husband in providing diabetic supervision and care so that he can take over on some evenings and let you relax a little. The second is that you do not give all your time and attention to your diabetic child. The other children and your husband need you too.

A last word to fathers

Careful research some years ago in my clinic showed that mothers were carrying the greater share of responsibility in caring for their diabetic children — and that almost half of them showed clear signs of strain. Fathers too often took the traditional view (not confined to Scotland) that their function was to beget children and to maintain them by the sweat of their brow. The mother's function was to bear the children and to care for them 24 hours each day. The old adage that a woman's work is never done was extended to understanding and dealing with diabetes.

There is less sweat on more brows nowadays and many mothers are themselves contributing to the family income. This diabetic care business should be shared and neither parent should duck his or her responsibility. Please help your wife, your child and the rest of the family. You may take your turn at child-minding so that your wife can relax for an evening. You may take the family out at weekends since the other children should not be deprived because of a brother's or sister's diabetes. You should certainly know about your child's food, insulin and exercise. Remember — 'for better or for worse, for richer or for poorer, in sickness and in health'. Father can give a special quality of strong support and leadership to the diabetic child.

A last word to both parents

Please remember that your diabetic child's future depends very much on *your* health. Your doctor knows that he can prescribe insulin, recommend diet and talk about exercise until he is blue in the face — *but*, if the supervising parent is physically ill or emotionally disturbed, it may all be in vain. If you have reason to believe that you are too sick, too tired or too troubled with your nerves to provide for your child please tell your doctor. He *is* interested and he may be able to help.

APPENDIX 1
YOUNG DIABETICS

Sugar diabetes (diabetes mellitus)

Sugar Diabetes in children is due to lack of insulin, the hormone essential to the production of energy from glucose. There is no danger in having a diabetic child in class. Few of them differ noticeably from other pupils. Almost all have insulin by injection before breakfast each day and many have a further injection before the main evening meal. Insulin keeps their blood glucose (sugar) level as normal as possible. If meals are delayed or the child has been unusually energetic the level may fall too low and the brain's supply of energy becomes inadequate for its normal function.

Symptoms

1. Hypoglycaemia, i.e. low blood glucose level or 'insulin reaction':

Mild	Moderate	Severe
Feels hungry	Emotional	Slumps or falls
Dizzy or faint	Thinks poorly	Resists help
Pale or flushed	Unsteady	Very confused
Skin moist	Heart rapid	Loses
Tremor	Eyes wander	consciousness
		Convulses (rare)

Symptoms can develop without warning in an apparently well diabetic child although others recognise them and seek help. It is a common problem in some but not in all diabetic children. Even if consciousness is lost there is no danger to life.

2. Ketoacidosis, i.e. high blood glucose level and insulin lack:

Thirst, increased frequency of passing urine (leaving class), weight loss, looks ill, deep breathing (as after running) and slow loss of consciousness over hours, breath smells sweet due to acetone (nail varnish remover).

Symptoms develop over many hours or days. Caring parents easily recognise it from urine tests.

Teachers can recognise it in the child of non-caring parents and this can be life-saving.

Treatment

1. Hypoglycaemia:

Mild	child should eat a snack or sweet (may carry such).
Moderate	adult make a solution of glucose (table sugar is effective but slower) and help the child to take it in small sips.
Severe	get nursing or medical help or, if this is not quickly available, call ambulance and transfer to hospital (doctor or nurse may give an injection of the hormone glucagon).

2. Never send a child with symptoms to his home unaccompanied.

3. Ketoacidosis:

Inform school doctor or nurse immediately so that the parents can be contacted and tests made.

Prevention

1. Ensure you have easy access to glucose or, less satisfactory, sugar if you have a diabetic pupil.

2. Make sure the diabetic child eats at the right times (check with school doctor/nurse).
3. Do not impose detention as a punishment unless he has a snack and unless the parents know he will be late home (they may fear he is unconscious somewhere).
4. Ensure that fresh fruit, ice cream, or biscuits and cheese are substituted for very sweet or steamed puddings at school meals.
5. Keep an eye on him in the swimming pool.
6. Encourage sport but ensure he has a snack before a mid-afternoon game — and a little extra at half-time.
7. Discourage smoking, alcohol, etc.
8. Ensure that the school tuck-shop (if such a facility exists) stocks low-calorie drinks suitable for diabetics and for the obese. Possibly encourage the neighbouring tuck-shop to do likewise.
9. Take him on school camps*, etc, if some member of staff is adequately briefed on care.

There are international stars in many sports who have been diabetic since childhood. In the gymnasium diabetic children are most unlikely to fall from ropes, etc. If feeling hypoglycaemic they will not climb.

Diabetic children can work as hard (physically and mentally) as others. They must not be over-protected and should be subject to the same disciplinary measures as their peers. Career guidance is important.

* The British Diabetic Association runs educational summer camps for diabetic children aged 8-12 years where good management is taught. The Association has also entered the field of adventure camps for adolescent diabetics (14-18 years) where they are taught how to cope with self-care under more challenging conditions.

APPENDIX 2

CARBOHYDRATE EXCHANGE LIST

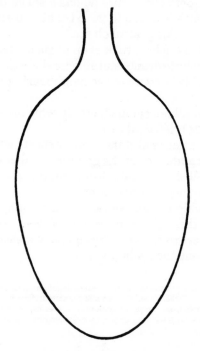

SIZE OF TABLESPOON USED IN COMPILING LIST

Further information may be obtained from the BDA.

© 1971 by the British Diabetic Association, 10 Queen Anne St., London W1M 0BD
Printed by F. J. Parsons (Westminster Press Ltd.), London and Hastings

CARBOHYDRATE EXCHANGE LIST

In view of metrication, weights of foods are given in GRAMS OF WEIGHT calculated as follows:

30 grams weight = 1 ounce
15 grams weight = ½ ounce
10 grams weight = ⅓ ounce

Liquid measures are expressed in MILLILITRES:

600 millilitres = 1 pint
300 millilitres = ½ pint
200 millilitres = ⅓ pint
150 millilitres = ¼ pint

Each of the following contains about **10 Grams Carbohydrate**

BREAD

			Metric grams (weight)
Brown or white	plain or toasted	½ slice of thick cut sliced large loaf	20
		⅔ slice of a thin cut sliced large loaf	20
		1 slice of a small sliced loaf	20

CEREAL FOODS

			Metric grams (weight)
Allbran		5 level tablespoons	25
Biscuits	plain or semi-sweet	2 biscuits	15

Each of the following contains about **10 Grams Carbohydrate**

CEREAL FOODS (continued)			**Metric grams (weight)**
Chappatis	made from wheat flour	1 level tablespoon	15
Cornflakes or other unsweetened breakfast cereal		3 heaped tablespoons	10
Cornflour	before cooking	2 heaped teaspoons	10
Cornmeal		1 level tablespoon	15
Custard powder	before cooking	2 heaped teaspoons	10
Flour		1 level tablespoon	15
Macaroni	before cooking	1 heaped tablespoon	15
Noodles	before cooking	1 heaped tablespoon	15
Porridge	cooked with water	4 level tablespoons	120
Rice	before cooking	2 heaped teaspoons	10
Rice	boiled	1 heaped tablespoon	30
Ryvita		1½ biscuits	15
Sago	before cooking	2 heaped teaspoons	10
Semolina	before cooking	2 heaped teaspoons	10
Spaghetti	before cooking	1 heaped tablespoon	15
Tapioca	before cooking	2 heaped teaspoons	10
Vitawheat		2 biscuits	15

MILK

			Metric millilitres
Milk	fresh or sterilised	14 tablespoons	200
Milk powder (skimmed)	reconstituted according to directions on tin	14 tablespoons	200
Milk	condensed, sweetened	1½ tablespoons	20

Each of the following contains about **10 Grams Carbohydrate**

MISCELLANEOUS FOODS

			Metric grams (weight)
Black pudding			65
Haggis			50
Haslet			60
Honey		2 level teaspoons	15
Jam		2 level teaspoons	15
Jelly	in packet, as purchased	1 small square	15
Ice cream	plain non dairy	1 small cornet or 1 small brickette	50
Lemon curd		2 level teaspoons	15
Marmalade		2 level teaspoons	15
Oatcakes			15
Polony			70
Potato bread			30
Potato scones			30
Pumpernickel			20
Sausages	full size	2 sausages, cooked	80
Sausages	chipolatas	4 chipolatas, cooked	80
Syrup		2 level teaspoons	15
Treacle		2 level teaspoons	15
Yoghurt	plain	1 carton	150

Sugar

To be used in an emergency, or sparingly in cooking. Do not use for sweetening tea or coffee or for sprinkling on fruit, cereals, etc, except when necessary in times of illness.

		Metric grams (weight)
Glucose	2 heaped teaspoons	10
Sugar	2 heaped teaspoons	10

103

Each of the following contains about **10 Grams Carbohydrate**
VEGETABLES (continued)

			Metric grams (weight)
Beetroots	boiled	3 heaped tablespoons	100
Carrots	boiled	4 heaped tablespoons	230
Corn	on the cob	1/2 large cob	80
Lentils	boiled	2 level tablespoons	60
Onions	fried	2 1/2 heaped tablespoons	100
Parsnips	boiled	2 heaped tablespoons	80
Peas	canned garden	4 heaped tablespoons	140
	fresh boiled	4 heaped tablespoons	130
	tinned processed	2 heaped tablespoons	70
	frozen boiled	7 heaped tablespoons	230
Plantains	boiled, steamed	1 1/2" section	30
Potatoes	boiled or jacket	1 the size of an egg	50
	chips	4 large chips	25
	crisps	1 level teacup	20
	mashed	1 heaped tablespoon	60
	roast	1 small	40
Sweet corn	tinned	2 level tablespoons	45
Sweet potato	boiled	2 level tablespoons	50
Yam	boiled	2 level tablespoons	35

Other vegetables and salads not on this list may be eaten without restriction.

BEVERAGES

		Metric grams (weight)
Bengers food	2 heaped teaspoons	15
Bournvita	2 heaped teaspoons	15
Horlicks	2 heaped teaspoons	15
Ovaltine	2 heaped teaspoons	15

		Millilitres
Coca-cola or Pepsi-cola		95

MILK (continued)

Milk			Metric milli-litres
Milk	evaporated, unsweetened	6 tablespoons	80

FRUIT
Stewed fruits should be cooked without sugar

			Metric grams (weight)
Apples	raw with skin and core	1 medium	100
	baked with skin	1 medium	120
	stewed	6 tablespoons	120
Apricots	fresh with stones stewed	3 large	190
	fresh with stones, raw	3 large	160
	dried, raw	6 halves	25
	dried, stewed	6 halves	60
Bananas	ripe without skin	1 small	50
Cherries	raw with stones	20	100
	stewed with stones	3 tablespoons	120
Currants	dried	1 level tablespoon	15
Damsons	stewed with stones	10	140
Dates	with stones	2	20
	without stones	3	15
Figs	green, raw	1 large	100
	dried, raw	1	20
	dried, stewed	1	35

FRUIT (continued)

Stewed fruits should be cooked without sugar

			Metric grams (weight)
Grapes	whole	10	60
Greengages	raw with stones	4	90
	stewed with stones	4	105
Nectarines	with stones	2	90
Oranges	without peel	1 large	120
Peaches	fresh with stones	1 medium	130
	dried, raw	2 halves	20
	dried, stewed	2 halves	50
Pears	raw with skin and core	1 medium	130
	stewed	2½ halves	125
Pineapple	fresh, edible part	2 heaped tablespoons diced	85
Plums	any dessert variety, raw with stones	3 large	110
	stewed with stones	5 medium	210
Prunes	dry, raw with stones	4 medium	30
	stewed with stones	4 medium	50
Raisins	dried	1 level tablespoon	15
Raspberries	raw	6 heaped tablespoons	180
Strawberries	fresh, ripe	15 large	160
Sultanas	dried	1 level tablespoon	15
Tangerines	without peel	2	120

Each of the following contains about **10 Grams Carbohydrate**

FRUIT (continued)

Stewed fruits should be cooked without sugar

			Metric milli- litres
Grapefruit juice	tinned, unsweetened	9 tablespoons	125
Orange juice	fresh or tinned, unsweetened	8 tablespoons	110
Pineapple juice	tinned, unsweetened	6 tablespoons	90
Tomato juice	tinned		285

The following contain a small quantity of Carbohydrate, and may be eaten in moderate quantity without being counted in the diet.

Avocado Pear, Blackberries, Blackcurrants, fresh Coco-nut, Grapefruit, Gooseberries, Lemon, Loganberries, Melon, Redcurrants, Rhubarb, Whitecurrants.

Each of the following contains about **10 Grams Carbohydrate**

NUTS (Shelled)	Metric grams (weight)
Almonds	230
Barcelona nuts	200
Brazil nuts	250
Chestnuts	30
Hazel nuts	150
Peanuts	120
Walnuts	200

VEGETABLES			Metric grams (weight)
Beans	baked, tinned	4 level tablespoons	95
	broad, boiled	2 level tablespoons	140
	butter, boiled	2 level tablespoons	60
	haricot, boiled	2 level tablespoons	60

APPENDIX 3

EMERGENCY RATIONS

A little wasted food, should an emergency ration prove to have been unnecessary, is a small price to pay for peace of mind during the journey. Eating arrangements at some of the world's airports may be primitive by day and virtually absent at night when a delayed flight makes a transit stop.

If such a place should offer a snack-bar or cafeteria (and those would be rather flattering descriptions for some of them) then freshly-cooked hens' eggs, fries, grills, toast, fresh chappatis, nuts and fruit with undamaged skin are usually safe. Cold meat and fish, salad and rice that looks to have lain cooked and exposed for a bit, ice-cream and ice should be avoided.

It is therefore reassuring to have with you at least half a day's rations i.e. for an 8 year old having 18 exchanges (180 g) of carbohydrate, take 9 extra exchanges if you are feeding him airline meals on board and a total of 27 if you are not. Since you are packing emergency rations and not a royal banquet the exchanges should be compact although a little variety is needed. Here are the basic components. Consult Appendix 2 (B.D.A. Exchange List for Diabetics) in which you will find the weight of each thing listed below providing 10 g. of carbohydrate.

Bread brown (wholemeal preferred) or white, sliced and buttered as sandwiches. These may be prefilled with protein foods such as meat, tinned fish, thinly spread peanut butter, cheese, egg or salad. Some may have a carbohydrate filling such as jam or stoned dates.

Biscuits these are very useful and sustaining. They include Ryvita, Vitawheat and oat cakes. A large tube of spreading cheese or a jar of diabetic jam makes them more interesting.

Potato crisps small individual packets.

Nuts a wide variety is listed.

Fruit apples, bananas, oranges, stoned dates, dried apricots, raisins.

Some chocolate and boiled sweets.

Extra protein may be taken as hard-boiled eggs, very well cooked cold chicken legs, or hard cheese (e.g. cheddar). Do not take tins unless you have checked with airport security services that they will be allowed in the cabin (they could be explosive and a tin-opener could be an offensive weapon). Diabetic fruit squash (*not* cans of diabetic drinks for the same reason) and a supply of water sterilising tablets.

Many an old soldier would have been very happy if his Jungle-Pack or K-ration had included such variety — and it is for a brief period only.

Index

Abroad, facilities for diabetic, 92
Acetest tablets, 51
Air hunger, 2, 63
Air travel precautions, 88
Alerting systems, 60–61
Alcohol, 85

BM-Test-Glycemie 20–800, 57
Breath in diabetic, 1, 13, 63
Breathing in diabetic, 3, 13, 63
British Diabetic Association, 6, 42

Camps for diabetic children, 86, 99
Carbohydrate, 10, 38
   allowance, 44
   exchange, 40, 47, 48
      list, 100–107
Cataract, 73
Clinitest apparatus, 51
Cold, exposure to, 18
Colour vision, importance in urine
      testing, 54
Coma, diabetic, 13
Complications, 58–65, 69–75
Cookery, diabetic, 43
'Cures', 7

Dental decay, 70
Dextrostix, 56
Diabetes, cause, 4, 97
   inheritance factor, 5
   symptoms, 5, 97
Diabetic associations, 6
Diet, 37–48
   advice service, 46

Drinks, 47
Drip therapy, 4
Drug addiction, 85

Eating, 37–48
Educational problems, 67, 72
Emergency rations, 108
Exchanges (carbohydrates), 40, 47,
      48
   list, 100–107
Exercise, 13, 49, 85
Eye-sight, disturbed, 58, 72–73.

Fat, 9
   loss at injection sites, 71
Fertility in diabetics, 7
Fibre, dietary, 10
Food, 'exchanges', 40, 47, 48,
      100–107
   for diabetics, 37–48
   good food system, 38
   refusal, 78
   relation to diabetes, 8–18
Foodstuffs freely allowed, 42
Future for diabetic child, 69–75

Gangrene, 7
Glucagon, 62
Glucose, 10, 11
   blood level, 12
      tests for, 56
   for emergencies, 61
   testing for, 51, 55
Good food system, 38
Growth disorders, 72

Guar gum, 45
Gun injectors, 33, 35

HbAlc, 57
Heart disease, 75
Height charts, 14—17
Height-weight range, attention to, 85
Home care team, 6, 39, 67
Hospital treatment, 3, 4
  discharge from, 66
Hostels for diabetics, 83
Hypocount monitor, 56
Hypoglycaemia, 21, 58, 59, 97
  differentiation from ketoacidosis, 64
  feigned, 79
  prevention, 98
  treatment, 98
Hypoguard injector, 35

Identity discs for diabetics, 60
Infections, protection from, 84
Information systems in emergencies, 60
Injections, 31, 33—36
  sites, 32
    swellings at, 71
Insulin, 20—36
  administration, 31, 33
  expiry date, 27
  human, effects of insufficiency, 11
    manufacture in the body, 5, 11
  injection, 31, 33—36
    omission by children, 78
    sites, 32
    timing, 25
  pump, 24
  reactions, 58—62
    causes, 60
    precautions, 60
    symptoms, 59
    treatment, 61
  regular 20
  soluble, 20
  strengths, 26
  syringe, 27—30
  types, 20, 21, 24
Insurance, medical, for holidays, 89
Intravenous therapy, 3

Ketoacidosis, 62
  differentiation from hypo-glycaemia, 4
Keto-diastix, 51
Ketones, 1, 13, 63
  testing for, 51
Ketostix strips, 51
Kidney, diabetic, 73

Lactose, 9, 10
Lumps at injection sites, 71

Meals, refusal, 78
Medic-Alert, 60
Medi-gen, 61
Menstruation, 7
Minerals, 11
Motion sickness, 91

Needles, 30
Nerve damage, 74

Obesity, 18

Pancreas, 5
Parents, advice to, 95
Parents' Groups, 6
Periods, menstrual, in diabetics, 7
Pregnancy problems, 75
Protein, 9, 39

Retinopathy, 73

School, 67, 98
Skin cleansing for injection, 33
Smoking, 85
'Somogyi-ing', 64
SOS Talisman, 61
Sports, 7, 18, 49
Starches, 10
Sugar, 10, 38
  substitutes, 46
Sweetening agents, 46
Swimming, 7, 18
Syringe, 27—30
  care and maintenance, 35
  disposable, 30
  needle, 30
  sterilisation, 29

Teachers, advice to, 98
Teeth, decay, 70
  hygiene, 71, 85
Thirst, 12
Travel abroad, 92
  arrangements, 88—91
  surface, 90
  time zones, 89
Treatment, checking, 50—57
  in hospital, 3, 4

Urine, 13
  testing, 50—56
    falsification, 76
    interpreting results, 55

Visual handicap, 72
Vitamins, 11
Vomiting, 91

Weight, attention to, 85
  charts, 14—17